Nature's Magic

A Colouring Book of Healing Plants and Remedies

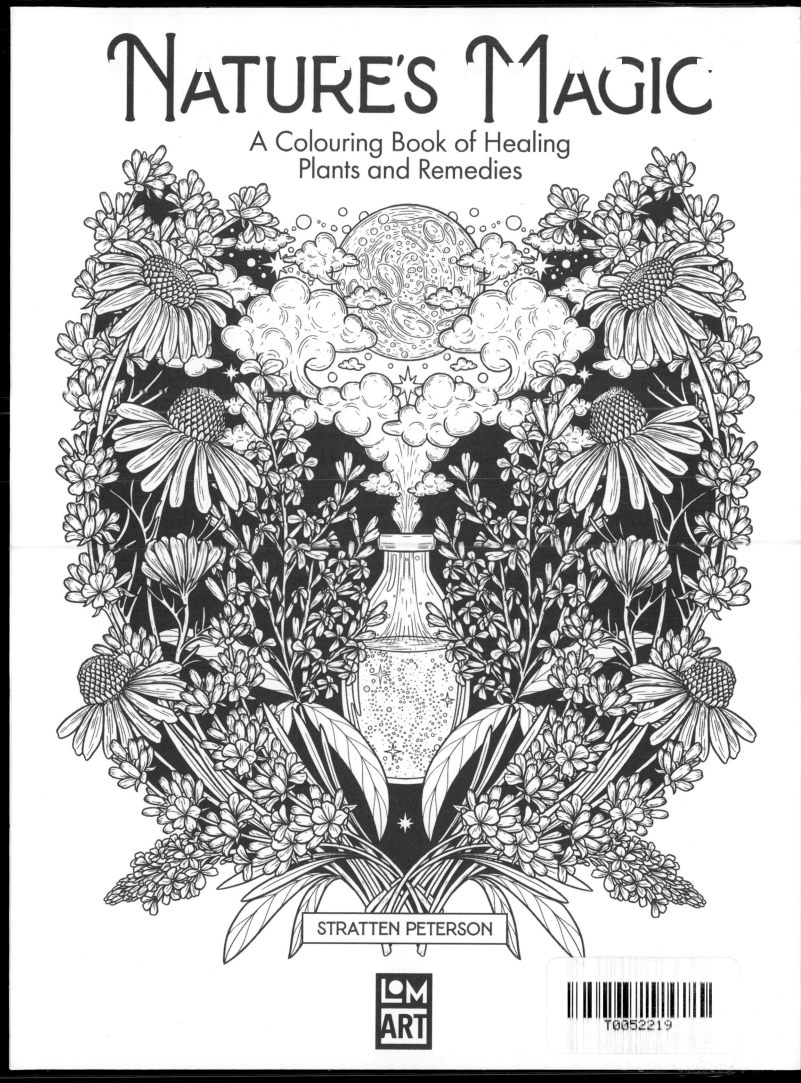

STRATTEN PETERSON

LOM ART

Illustrated by
Stratten Peterson

Written and edited by Imogen Currell-Williams
Designed by Jade Moore
Cover designed by Angie Allison

First published in Great Britain in 2023 by LOM ART, an imprint of Michael O'Mara Books Limited,
9 Lion Yard, Tremadoc Road, London SW4 7NQ

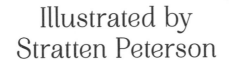

W www.mombooks.com/lom   f Michael O'Mara Books   ✗ @OMaraBooks   ◉ @lomart.books

A CIP catalogue record for this book is available from the British Library.

ISBN: 978-1-912785-95-7

1 3 5 7 9 10 8 6 4 2

This book was printed in China.

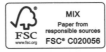

Disclaimer
This book is not a medical handbook and the ingredients
are not recommended for use. The publisher and author disclaim all
liability, as far as is legally permitted, for accidents or injuries or loss
of any nature that may occur as a result of the use or misuse
of the information and guidance given in this book.

Introduction

This beautiful compendium celebrates the wonder, wisdom and healing power of Mother Nature.

Inspired by traditional remedies and rituals, the detailed pictures in this book feature powerful combinations from nature's apothecary. The healing herbs, plants and flowers reflect the fascinating history and folklore behind their use.

Let nature inspire you as you complete the stunning artworks.

The Power of Protection

Used as an antidote to venomous animal bites, the concept of the 'theriac' first appeared in Greek mythology and has a rich history. Theriac comes from the Greek word *theria*, meaning wild beasts. Over time, it has been used to treat a huge variety of illnesses. With a list of ingredients developed by many physicians over the years, its use continued into medieval Europe, most notably in Italy, where it was known as the Venice Treacle.

Here, a twisted snake (a traditional pharmacy symbol) wraps itself around the elements of one of the earliest incarnations of theriac – thyme, sweet myrrh, aniseed, fennel and parsley.

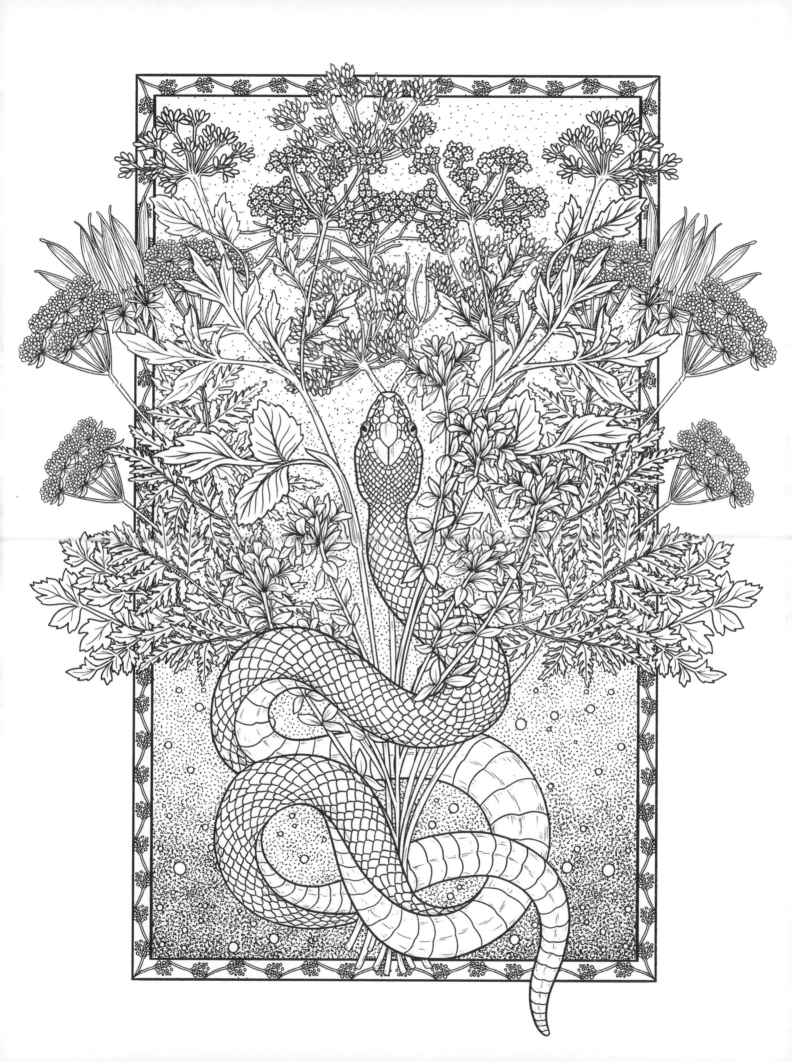

Digestive Aid

This ornate teacup is brimming with a restorative tea to improve digestion and soothe the stomach. Dandelion, ginger root, liquorice and peppermint bring the herbal qualities that are said to make this tea so effective. The luscious green leaves are interspersed with golden dandelions, purple and white mint flowers and the bright red flowers of the ginger plant.

The anti-inflammatory properties of ginger and liquorice can help to reduce sickness, cramping and bloating. Dandelion serves as a bitter herb, which can promote digestion by stimulating the body's own digestive processes. Peppermint has similar qualities, as well as helping to relax the muscles in the digestive tract and adding a pleasing flavour and scent to the tea.

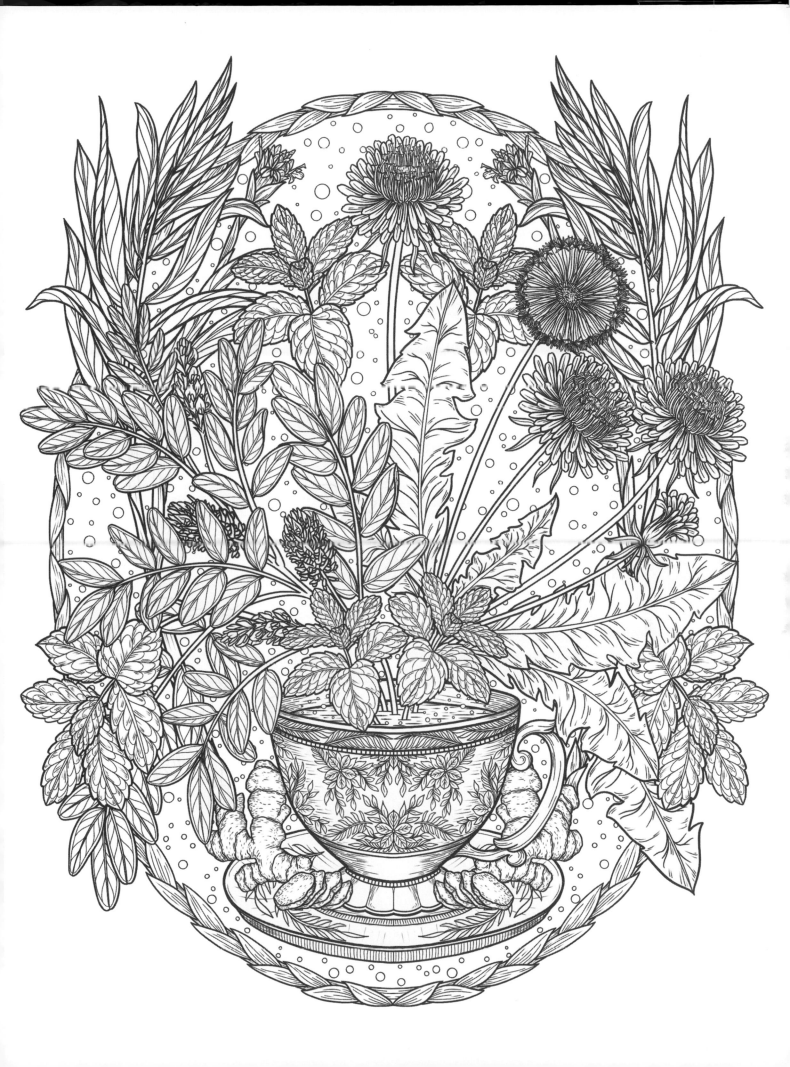

Sleeping Potion

Let the soothing qualities of lavender, chamomile
and verbena bring you a peaceful night's sleep
and a deep sense of relaxation and rejuvenation.

This small vial contains a powerful concoction of plants
with sleep-inducing qualities. Lavender has long been used for
its health benefits and, most helpful for this potion, it is thought
to support sleep, calm the nervous system and lift the mood.
Chamomile and purple verbena both aid relaxation and, when
paired with lavender, the scent is overwhelmingly calming.
For this reason, lavender is also often used as an essential
oil. The potion shown here diffuses its hypnotic scent
into the night sky and forms hazy clouds.

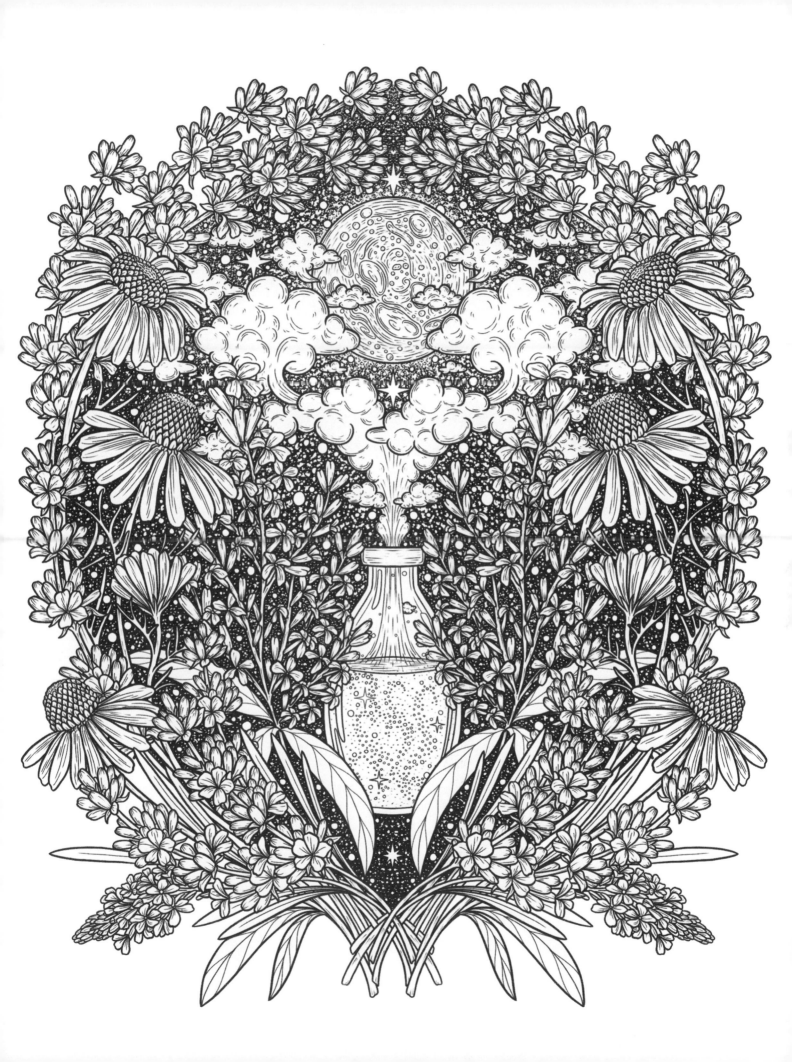

Nine Herbs Charm

The Nine Herbs Charm originates from an Anglo-Saxon
manuscript dating back to 1000 CE and was said to offer healing
and protection. It is made up of nine different herbs that were crushed
and mixed into a salve, which was then applied to the patient while
a charm was chanted. The nine herbs featured in this specific
incarnation are chamomile, mugwort, lamb's cress, plantain,
fumitory, nettle, crab apple, chervil and fennel.

Here, the scented flowers of white chamomile, pink fumitory,
pale yellow mugwort, white chervil and pink crab apple
are surrounded by leafy green herbs and
a Sun bursting with radiance.

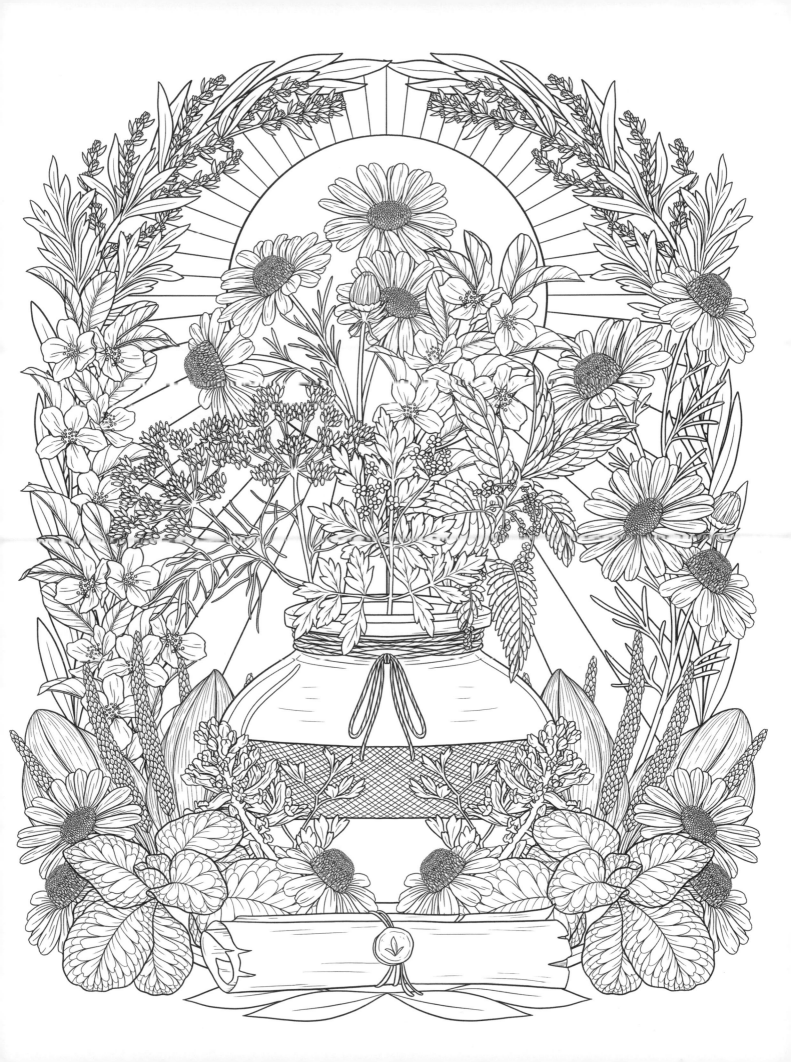

Potion to Ease the Heart

The hawthorn tree has a long-recorded history of medicinal use.
In the spring, it blossoms with white or pink flowers and in the colder
months it produces red berries, providing a haven for animals throughout
the year. The hawthorn is a member of the rose family, a group of plants
closely associated with the heart, and both its flowers and berries have
traditionally been used to treat heart ailments. An ancient Greek physician,
Dioscorides, recommended using hawthorn to increase blood flow to the
heart, and the tree was also used spiritually to heal a broken heart.

Here, a blackbird perches on a hawthorn branch, above its favourite
food, the berries. It is clutching the chain of a heart-shaped locket
in its beak, symbolizing the healing power this plant has.

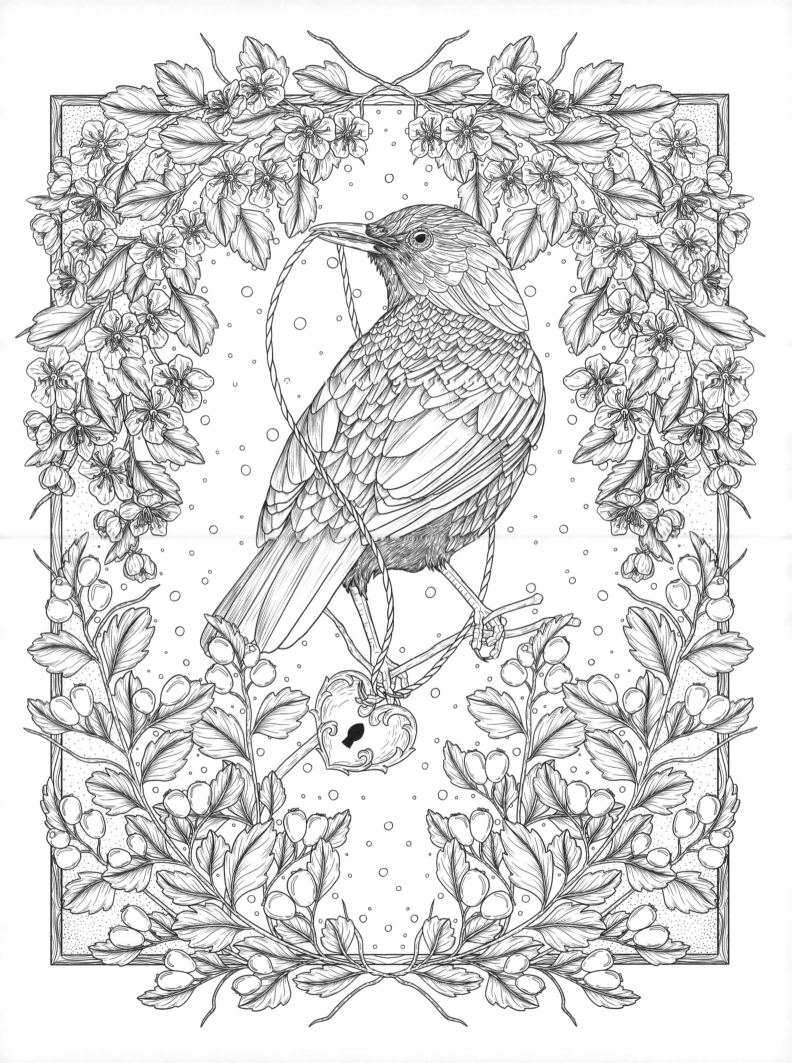

Moon Fruit Powder

The gardenia was commonly used in magic to attract love.
The flower has a strong, intoxicating scent, and its
thick petals contrast with its glossy dark green leaves.

The flowers were often called 'Moon fruit', due to their association
with Morpheus, the Greek god of dreams. The Greeks in particular prized
the scent of this bloom, believing it could transport them to paradise.
A popular recipe was to take the white petals, also called 'Moon's tears',
and leave them to dry in the Sun. Once they were dry, the petals were
ground into a fine powder in a pestle and mortar. This magical powder
was then brushed all over the body, while making a wish for love.

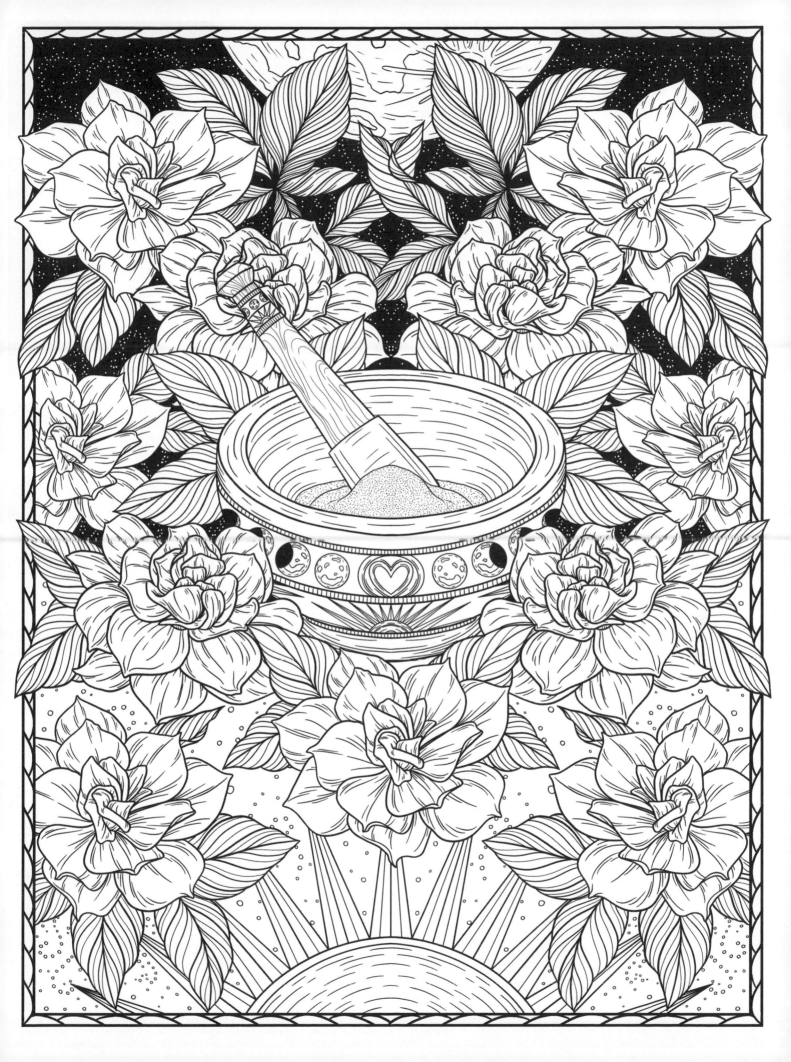

Turmeric Milk

Turmeric has been used for thousands of years as a potent
ingredient, for both food and healing. It originates from India and is
an integral part of Ayurvedic healing, the traditional system of medicine
used in India. It is believed that the benefits from this plant take place
deep inside our organs, reducing inflammation, allowing the liver to detoxify
itself and improving skin quality. Turmeric has an active ingredient called
curcumin, which has anti-inflammatory qualities that are said
to aid ailments, such as arthritis, allergies and infections.

The healing milk in this picture combines the power of turmeric
with cumin, black pepper, cinnamon sticks, ginger, star anise, vanilla
and agave. Each adds their own distinctive quality and flavour,
while aiding the absorption of the main ingredient – turmeric.

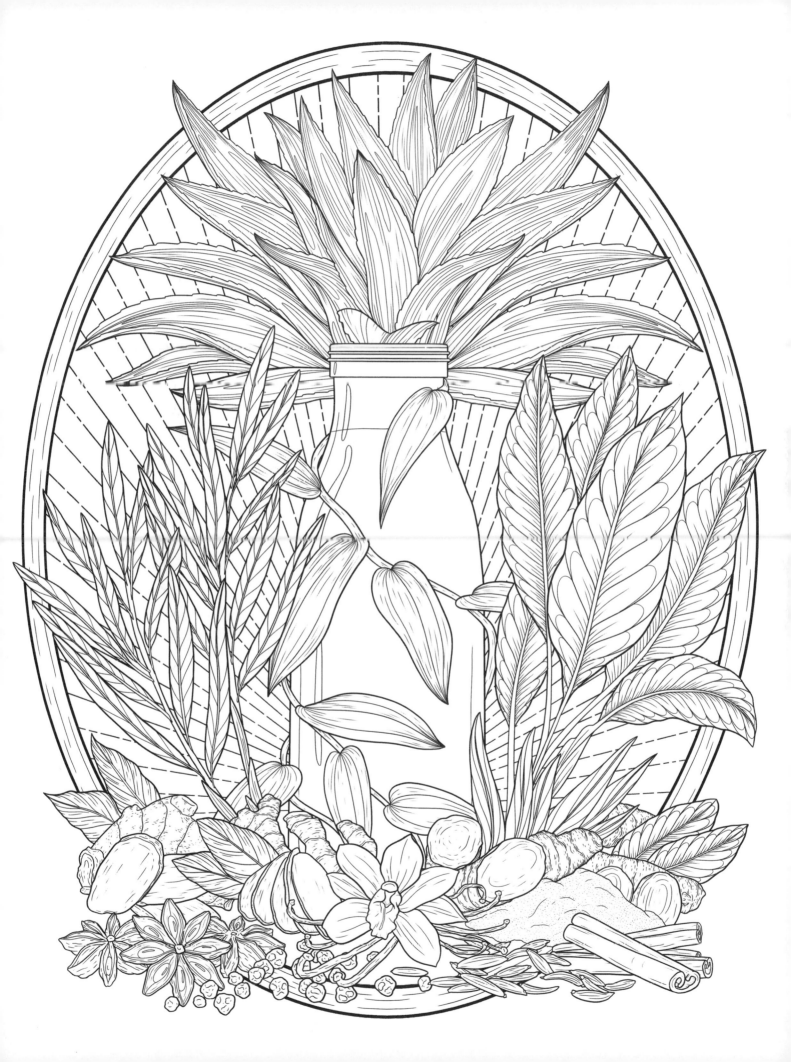

Banish Nightmares

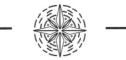

The peony is a beautiful and colourful bloom, with huge heads of petals that come in a variety of colours, from pale pastels to vibrant reds. In folklore, it was associated with the Moon's uplifting energy and thought to keep evil spirits at bay.

Medieval monks used peonies in a number of remedies. The seeds were considered to be particularly potent, and were often strung together and worn like a necklace for protection. One common sleep potion used 15 peony seeds, which were soaked in a goblet of wine or mead. The seeds were removed and the potion was taken at bedtime to banish nightmares. Here, the delicate blooms are contrasted with a starry night sky under a full moon, alongside an ornate goblet.

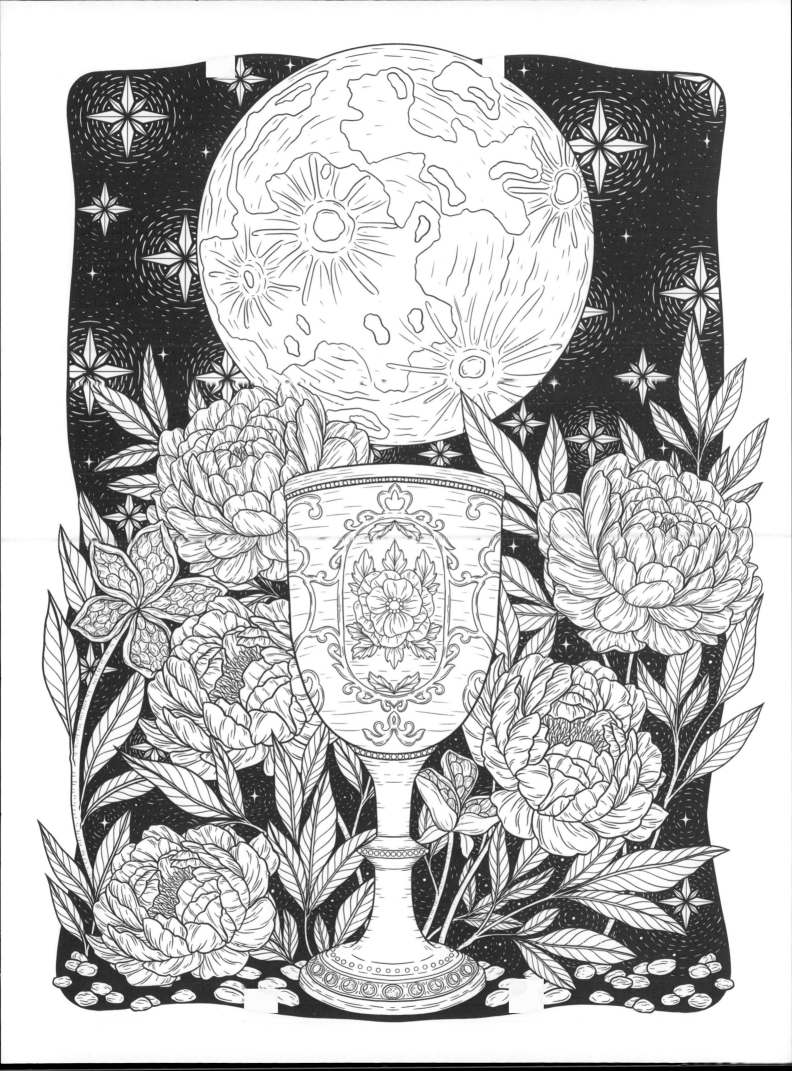

Healing Balm

Calendula plants have long been used in herbology. The rich orange flowers follow the Sun and radiate the nourishing energies they absorb, symbolized by the Sun rays in this image.

Here, the plant is mixed with purple lavender flowers to form a balm. Calendula petals are said to be anti-inflammatory and, when mixed with the calming and soothing benefits of lavender, create a healing balm that also has a restorative and aromatic scent. This balm has been used for centuries to heal wounds, treat stings and calm skin conditions. Even modern-day products feature calendula for its healing properties.

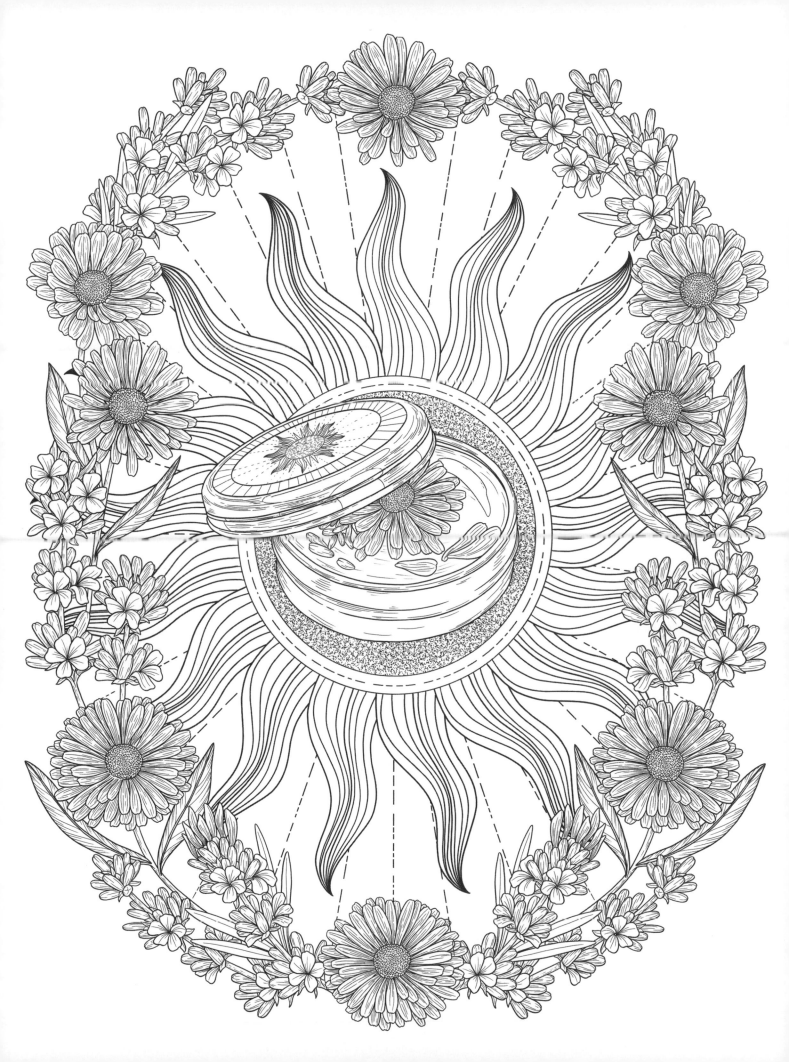

Remedy for Tired Eyes

Cornflower comes in a variety of colours, but is most commonly
a cool purple-blue colour. It has soothing qualities that can be used
to alleviate irritation of the eyes, sunburn and skin inflammation.

It is paired here with two other wildflowers, greater plantain,
with its long, straw-coloured flower spikes and eyebright, which
has white flowers tinged with purple. Greater plantain has historically
been used as an antihistamine and eyebright has been used for eye
infections and eye fatigue. This image reflects these plants' association
with tired eyes, with the delicate flowers creating eyelashes
surrounding an iris filled with petals.

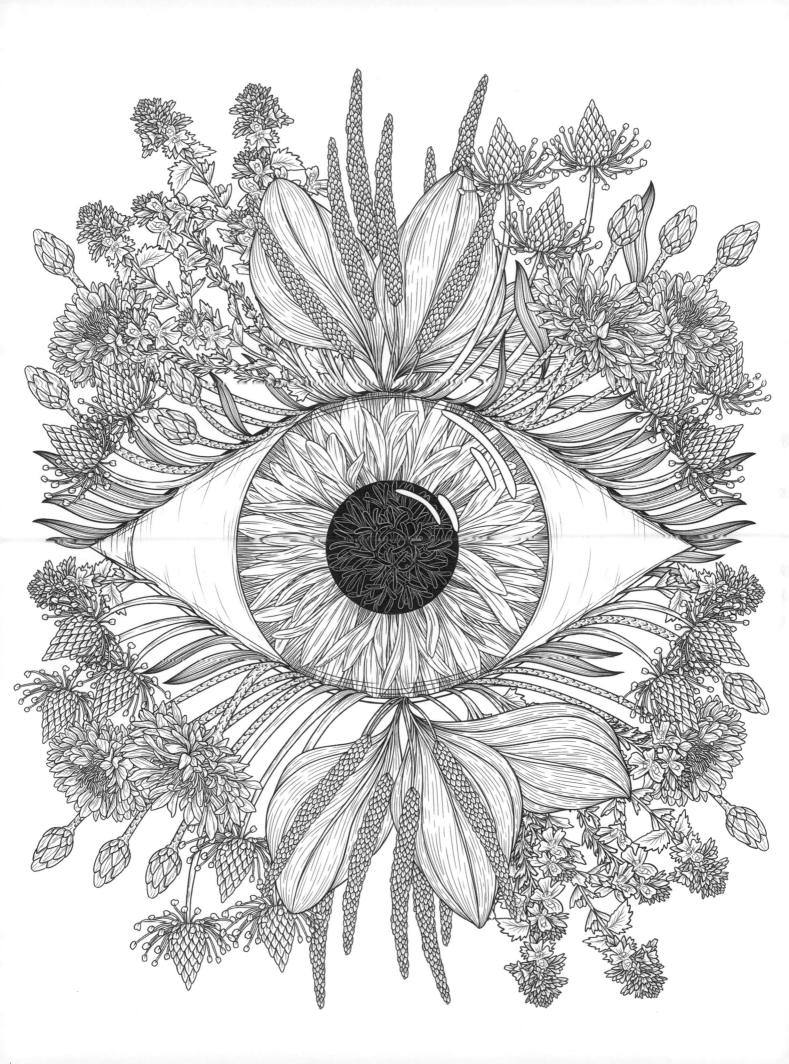

Plant of Immortality

Known as the 'plant of immortality' by the ancient Egyptians,
aloe vera has long been revered as a powerful and potent ingredient,
promoting health and wellness. It has been used for thousands of
years across the world to treat all manner of ailments, from
burns and wounds to soothing fevers. The ancient Egyptian
queens Cleopatra and Nefertiti are said to have used it
daily, and it is still largely used today for its benefits.

Here, succulent, green aloe plants with their distinctive red
flowers surround an ankh symbol, also known as the key of life.
This well-known hieroglyph is often shown in the hands of Egyptian
pharaohs and queens. An ankh amulet was often buried within
a sarcophagus and was seen as a symbol of life and immortality.

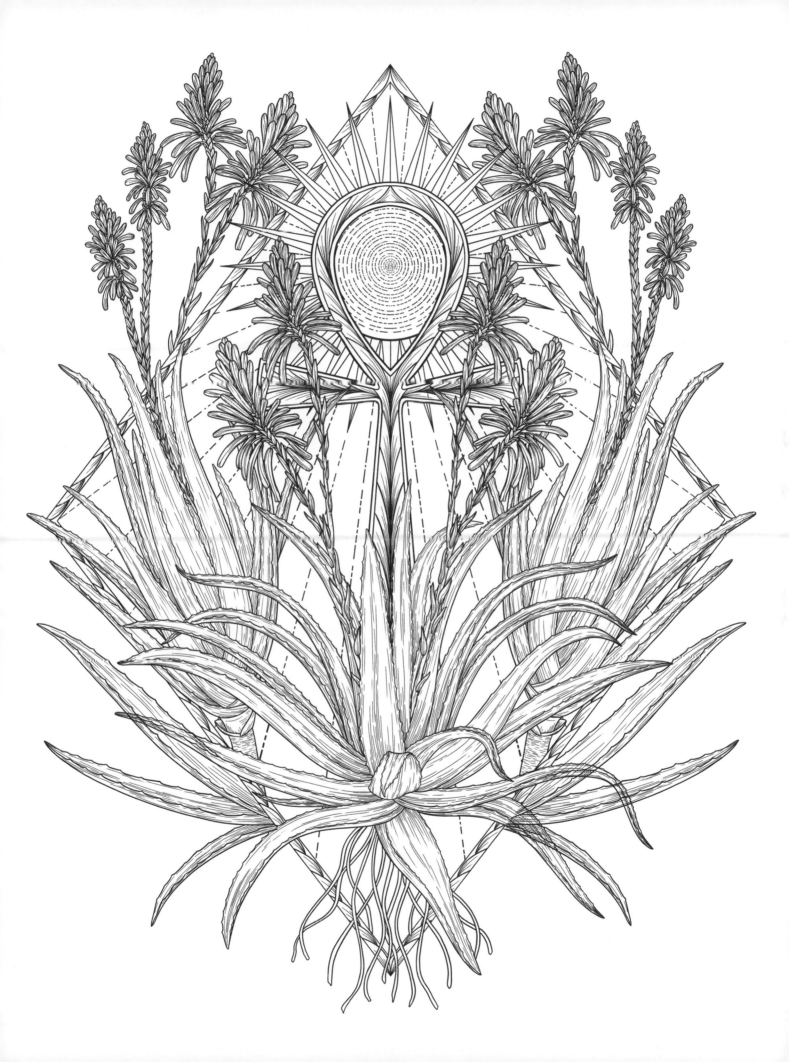

Acorn Amulet

In folklore, the acorn is a potent symbol synonymous with strength and protection. Sacred to the Druids, the acorn was believed to be imbued with the power of its parent tree, the oak. Wearing or carrying an acorn was thought to protect a person from thunder and lightning, and the nut was often used as magical charm for strength and personal power.

The Celts created charms by taking an acorn and washing it in fresh water. The nut was then left in the light of the full Moon for one night to infuse it with lunar energy. It could be carried all the time or held when someone needed extra strength. This illustration represents the protection acorns offer, alongside an aging oak tree.

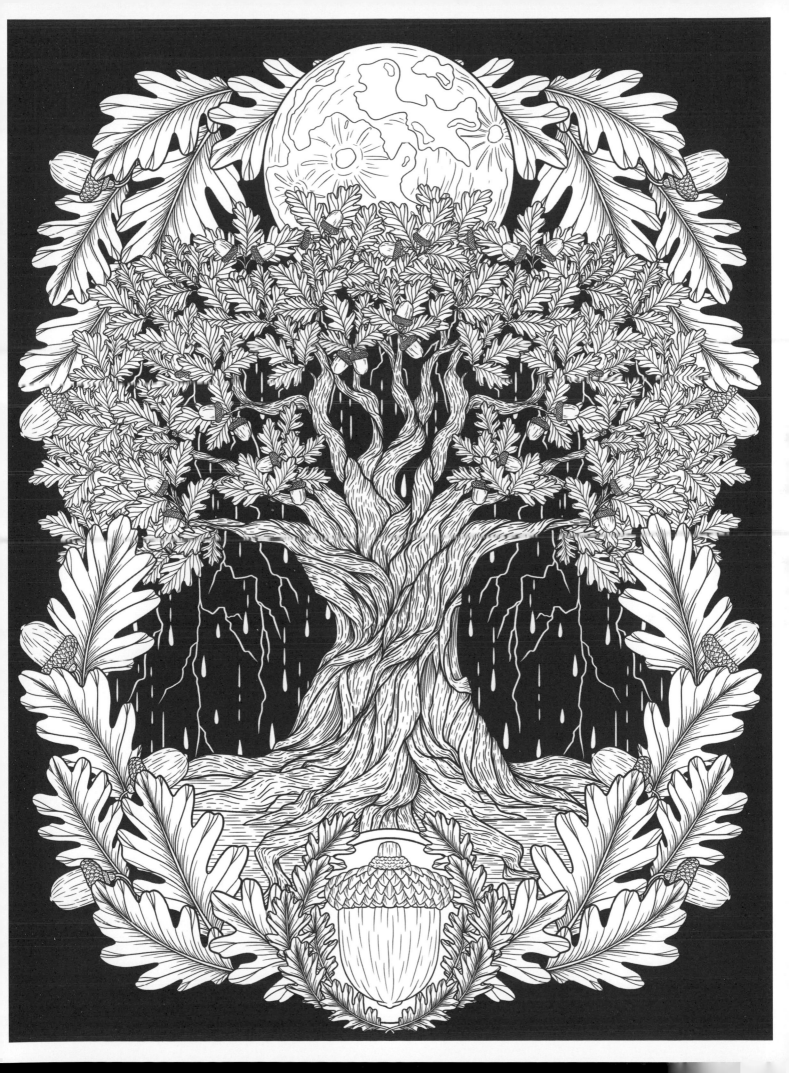

Prosperity Tea

This ornate teapot is brimming with plants that
are believed to bring abundance. Basil, nutmeg and
mint are surrounded by stacks of gold and jewels,
symbolizing bounty, prosperity and good fortune.

The green leaves of basil are lush and vibrant, with a
distinctive scent. In folk magic, this aromatic herb was thought
to attract good things, from love to prosperity. It was often used
to create a tea by boiling the leaves in water and straining it.
Honey was added to sweeten the taste. Nutmeg was known for
its ability to procure good luck and mint could be added
for those who wished for an abundance of love.

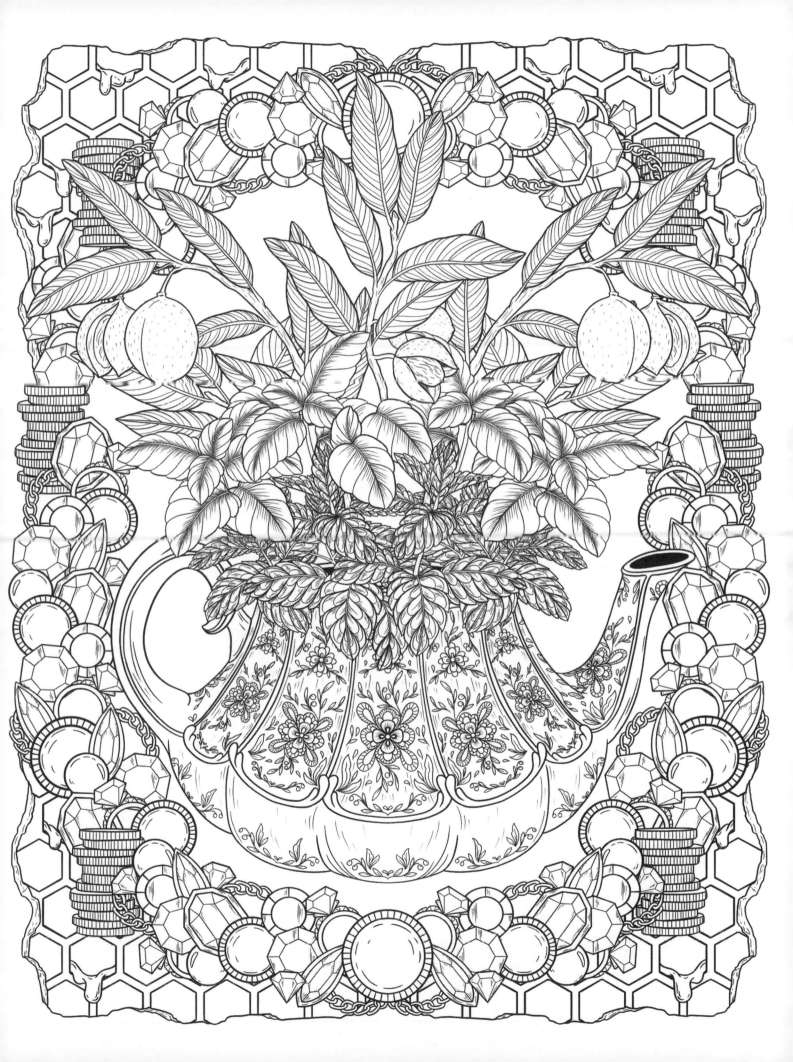

Sunshine Scent

The radiant sunflower is a symbol of joy and abundance.
The ancients believed this plant held positive energy, inspired by
the way the flowers naturally follow the path of the Sun (a phenomena
known as phototropism). This, along with its golden petals, makes the
sunflower a popular choice in magic to promote happiness, especially
if it is combined with other yellow and orange blooms. Here, it is
paired with pale yellow daffodils, which have a sweet scent,
and are believed to be a positive omen.

A magical fragrance was created by steeping petals from
both sunflowers and daffodils in hot water, leaving the mixture
to simmer for a long time, then decanting it into a vessel. The
water could be sprinkled around the home, and even dabbed
on to pulse points, like a perfume, to attract blessings.

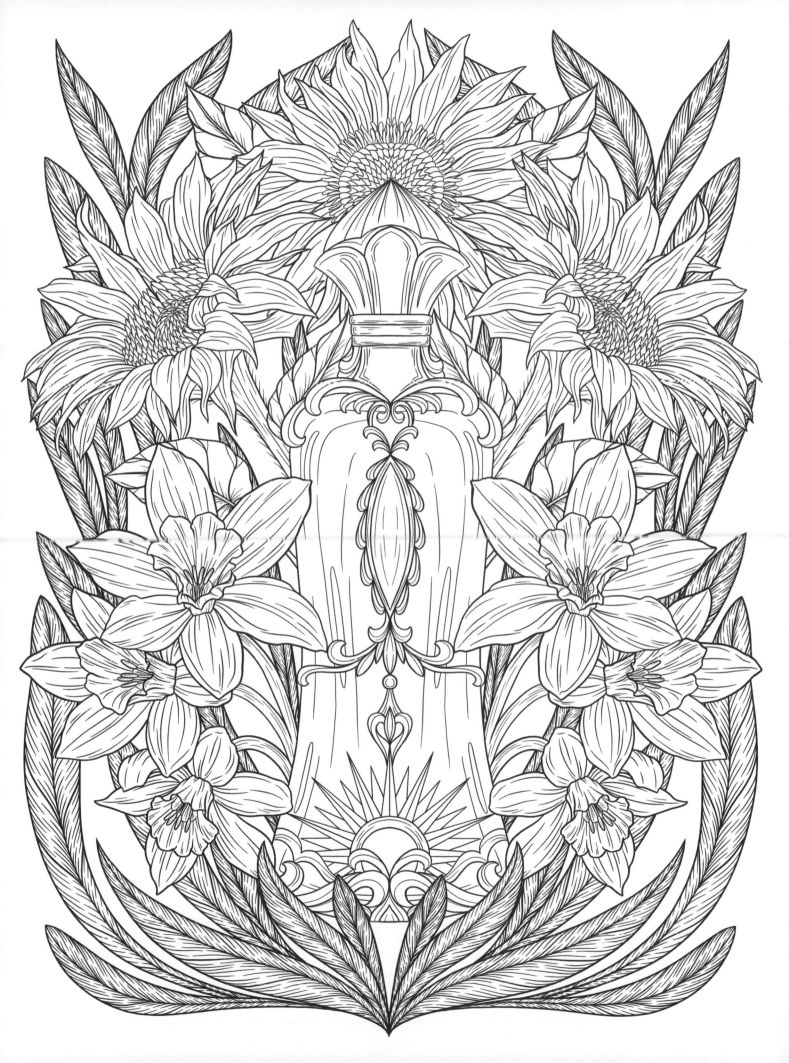

Healing Infusion

This beautiful pattern of camellias and monarch
butterflies represents a floral healing infusion, which
was used to make sweet-scented bathing water.

Traditionally, camellia flowers were associated with youth,
and extracts of the oil were rubbed into the skin. The petals
from the flowers, which are often pink or red, were considered
particularly powerful. Camellias are popular with the distinctive
orange-and-black monarch butterflies, who rest on the
flower heads. Butterflies have long been associated with
change and renewal, and just touching a butterfly's
wing was believed to grant the gift of immortality.

For this infusion, blooms that a butterfly had rested
upon were picked and soaked in warm water. Pink rose
petals were also added to enhance the potion with
the power of inner beauty and a delicate scent.

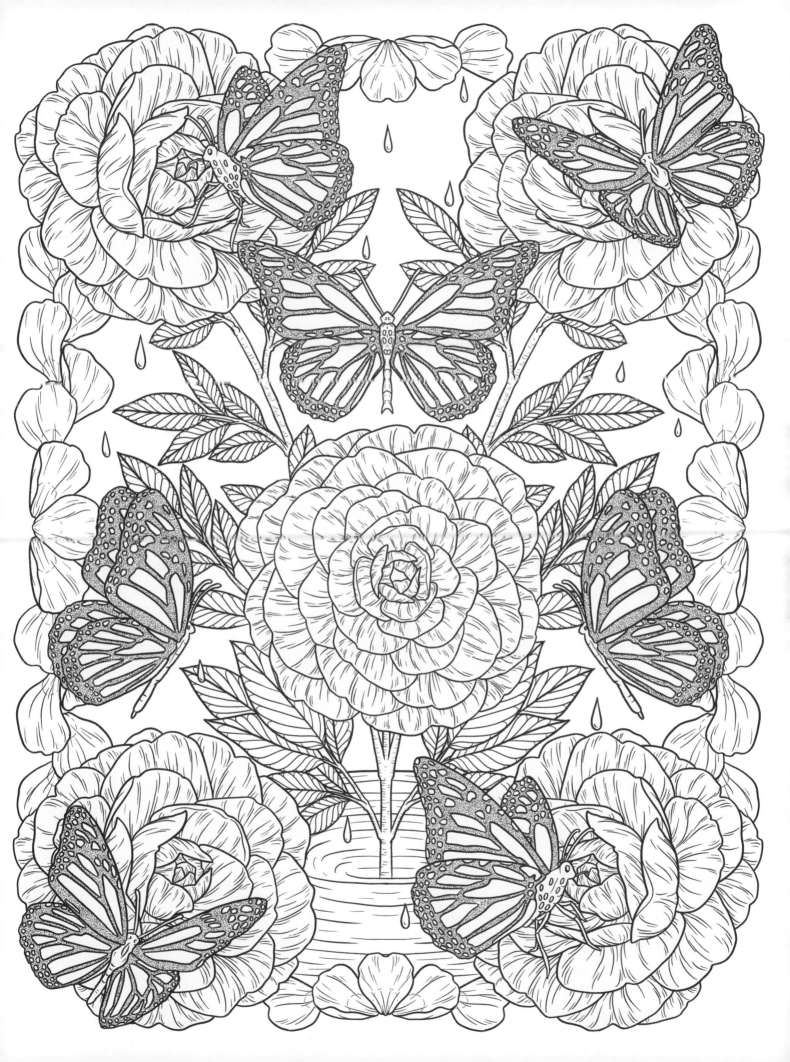

Scented Sachet

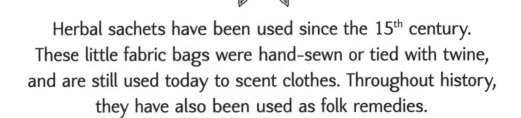

Herbal sachets have been used since the 15th century.
These little fabric bags were hand-sewn or tied with twine,
and are still used today to scent clothes. Throughout history,
they have also been used as folk remedies.

This sachet features cloves and benzoin, a sweetly scented resin,
mixed with bundles of thyme and sage. The pale green sage leaves
were renowned for their cleansing properties, which were enhanced
when paired with thyme. The strong scent of the deep brown cloves and
golden benzoin was believed to keep negative energy at bay. With these
four ingredients mixed together, this particular concoction was used
as an insect repellent and tied on a belt around the waist.

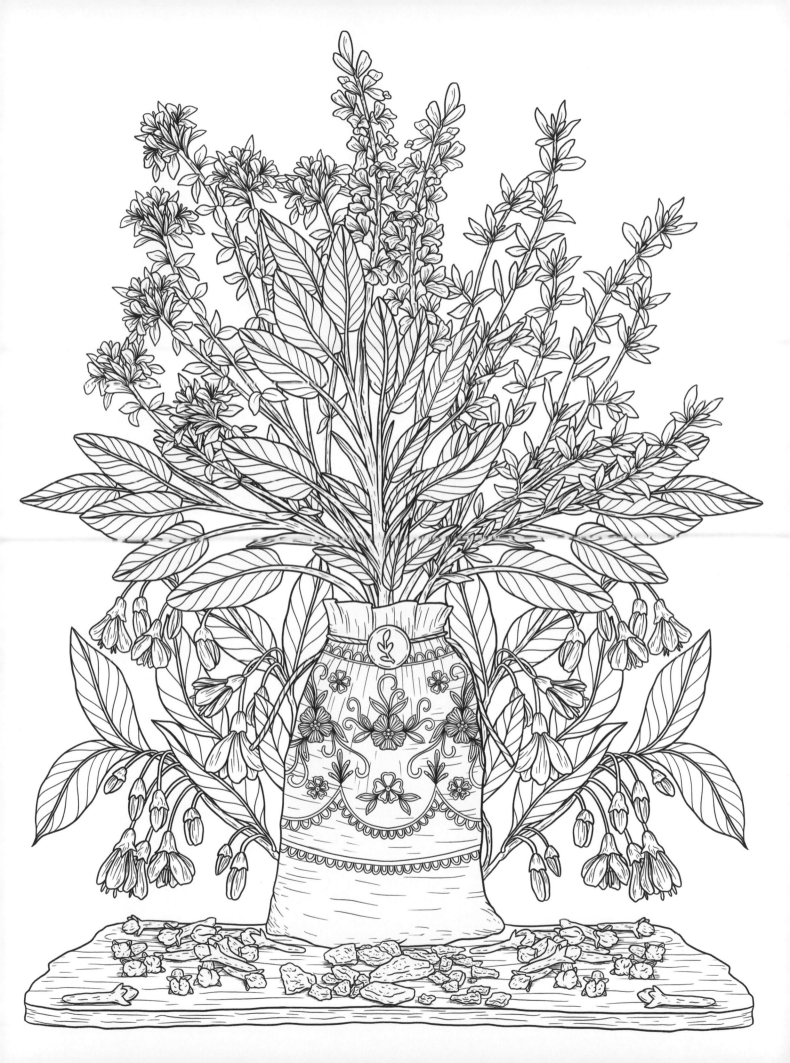

Youth Potion

Wild cherries have a long association with youth and beauty.
In folklore, they were considered a symbol for renewal. Ripening
on the tree, they were thought to represent the innocence of youth.
It was also believed that cuckoos needed to eat three good meals
of cherries before they could stop singing their distinctive song.

An infusion of rich red or black cherries along with the
bark from the wild cherry tree was made by boiling equal
amounts of the fruit and wood together, then decanting into
a bottle or jar. This was thought to cure ailments, and
give those who drank it vigour and vitality.

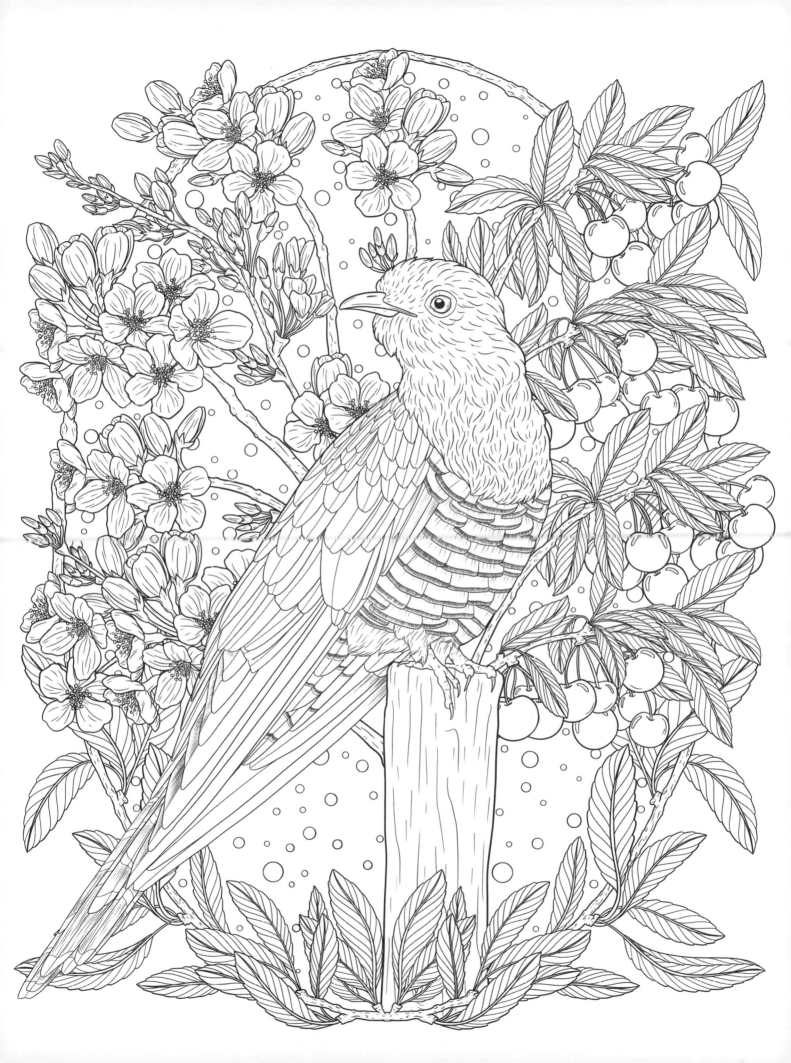

A Myriad of Mushrooms

Mushrooms have been consumed for their medicinal qualities
for many thousands of years. The first known reference is found in
an Ayurvedic source from 5000 BCE. There is also a Chinese compendium
of mushroom usage that dates back several thousands of years. In the
past, some of the rarest mushroom species were so expensive and so
hard to find that only Chinese emperors could eat them. The ancient
Greeks referred to mushrooms as food of the gods.

Mushrooms are believed to have qualities that provide immune support,
balance blood sugar and support the nervous system and brain
health, as well as being packed with vitamins and minerals.

The seven species of mushroom featured in this artwork represent
the visual diversity of the fungi kingdom, and range in colour from
white to vibrant orange. They are: chanterelle, king oyster,
cauliflower, honey fungus, shimeji, Caesar's and enoki.

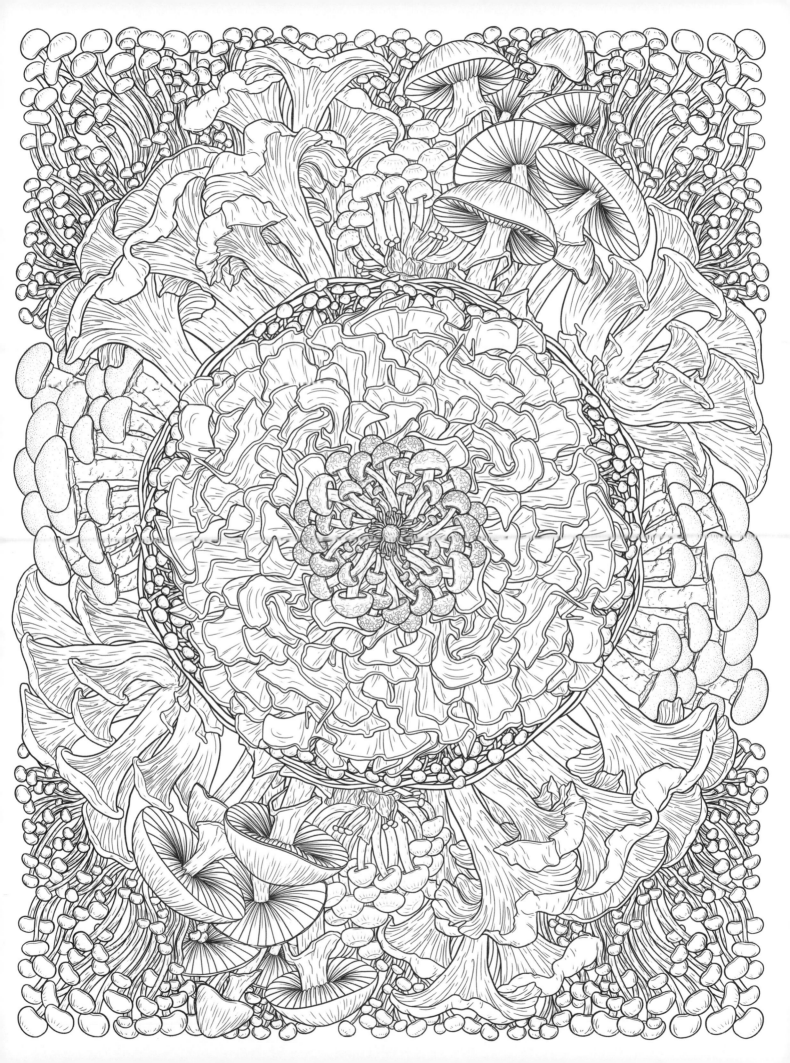

Blackberry Bramble

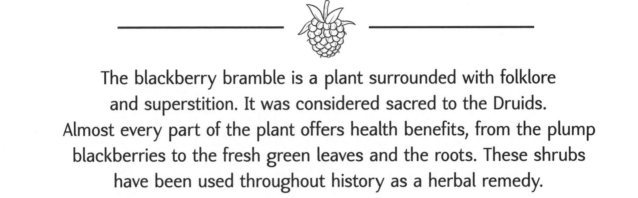

The blackberry bramble is a plant surrounded with folklore
and superstition. It was considered sacred to the Druids.
Almost every part of the plant offers health benefits, from the plump
blackberries to the fresh green leaves and the roots. These shrubs
have been used throughout history as a herbal remedy.

The berries themselves are a powerful source of antioxidants
and contain high levels of fibre, vitamin C and vitamin K. The plant
has historically been used to treat sore throats, mouth ulcers and gum
inflammations. It has also been made into compresses that were
used externally to heal wounds and bruises, as the tannins in
the leaves and roots are said to help control bleeding.

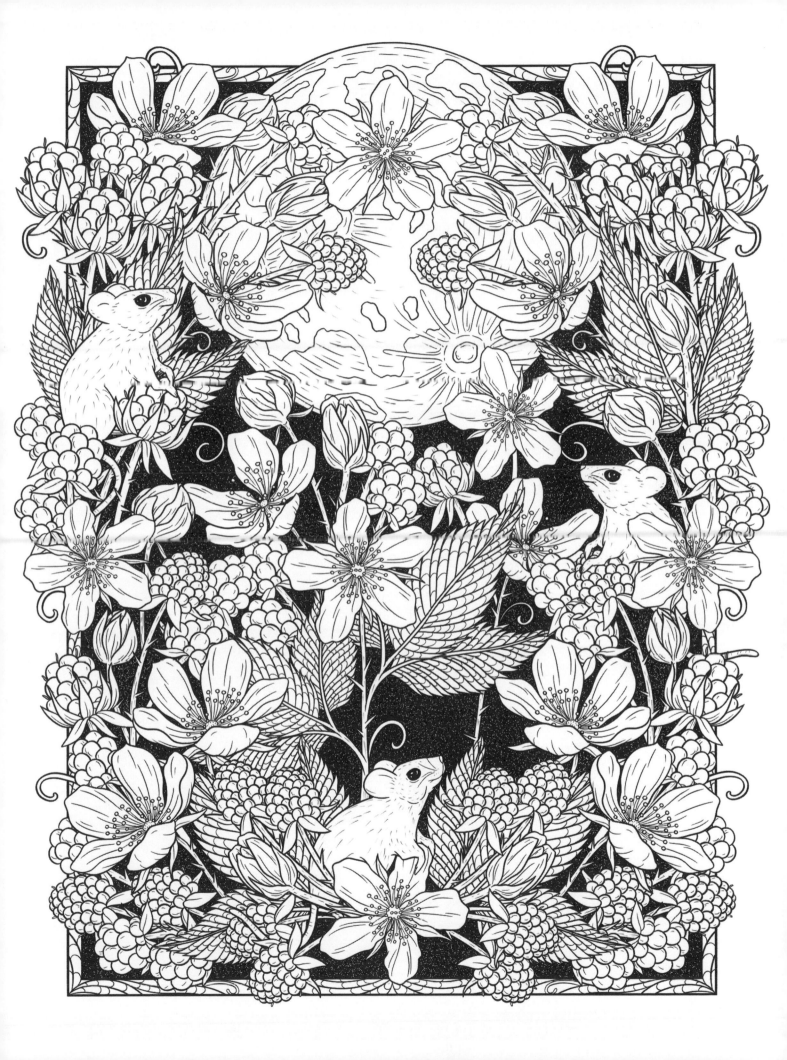

Ocean Remedy

This aquatic scene features an array of seaweed surrounding colourful ocean creatures. Seaweed is the common name for a variety of different species of algae that grow in oceans, rivers, lakes and other water bodies. Rich in vitamins and minerals, many species of seaweed have anti-inflammatory and antimicrobial properties and have featured in medicines around the world for thousands of years.

Seaweed was used by the ancient Greeks and Romans to treat wounds, burns and rashes, while ancient Chinese and Japanese medicine used the plants to treat glandular problems. Different seaweeds are used for different maladies. Most commonly today, it is a popular food item, largely consumed in Asia, but enjoyed around the world.

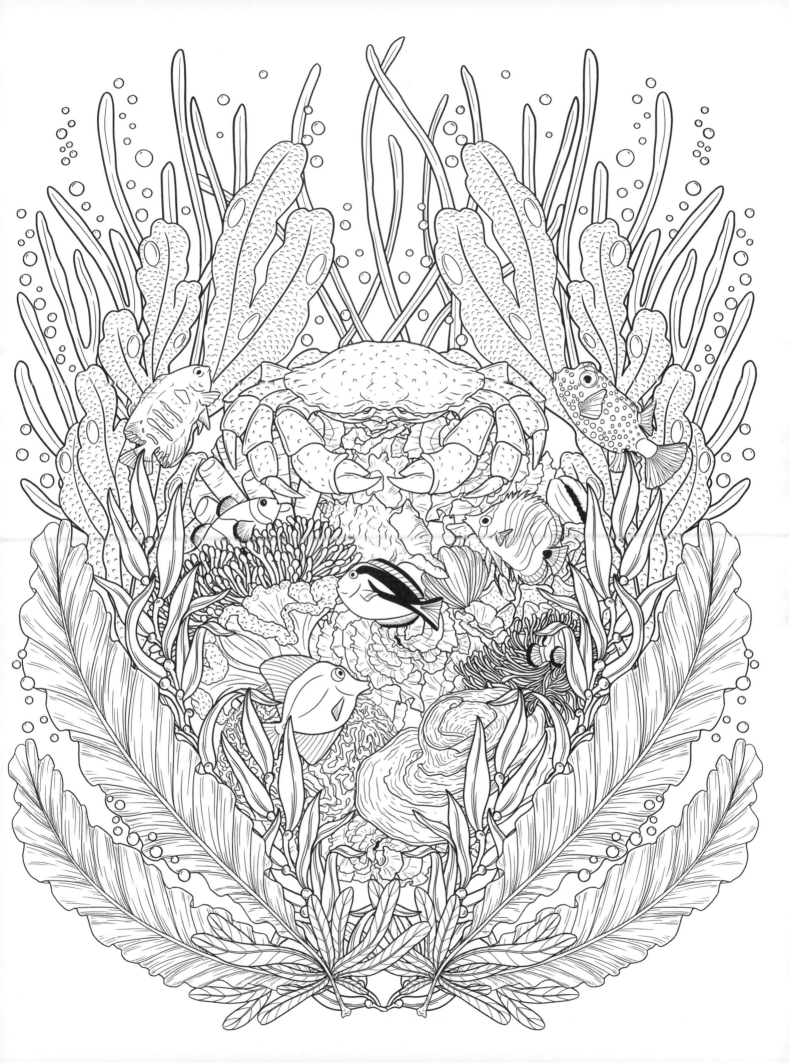

Vitality Tonic

Used in ancient Greece, Asia and in folk medicine for
thousands of years, the dandelion has a vast medicinal history.
Its use was even recorded in an ancient Chinese herbal manual
in 659 CE. Dandelions have long been used in folklore for divination,
and in herbal concoctions as a tonic for the body and mind.
With their fluffy seedheads, known as clocks, they're
a common sight in meadows and gardens.

A traditional tonic was made from the dried leaves and roots.
These were fermented in apple cider vinegar in a jar and stored
in a cool, dark place for over a month. The juice of a whole
lemon was then added and the tonic was complete. It was
dropped into other beverages or taken by itself.

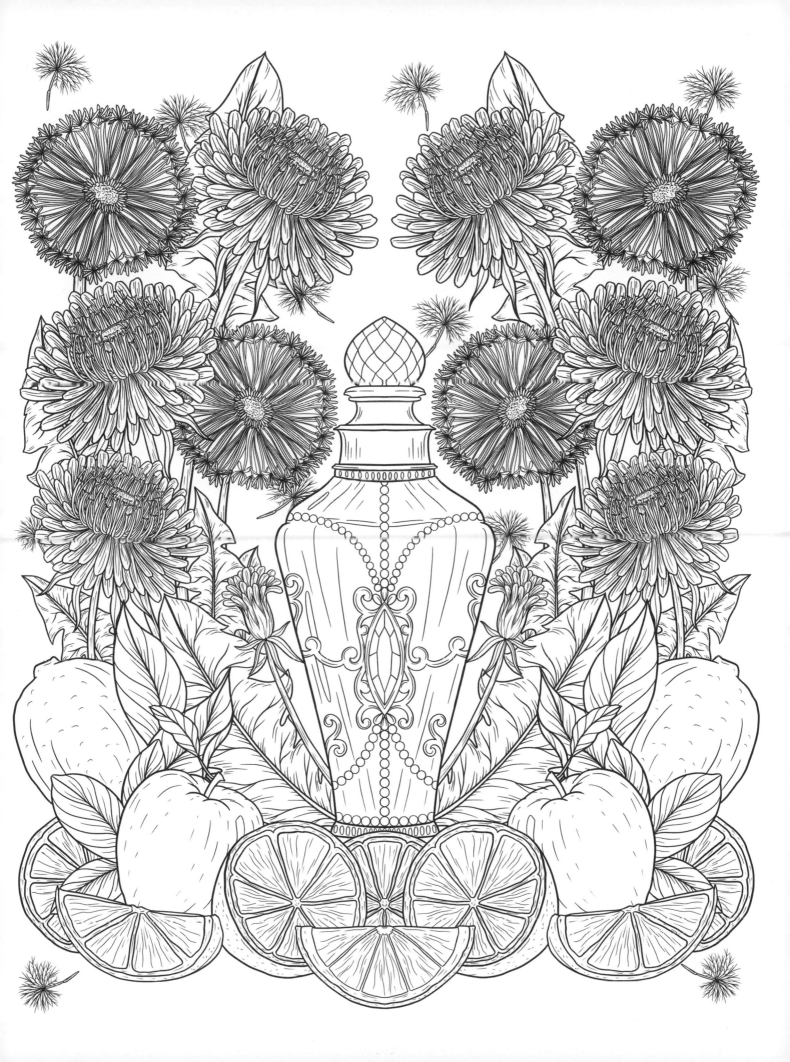

Tranquility Tincture

Valerian has long been considered a powerful herb. The Celts
used to hang bundles in their windows to prevent lightning
from striking their homes. In medieval times, the herb was
used in healing infusions to soothe and calm the mind.
The flowers come in a variety of colours, usually
pink or white and sometimes a deep red.

The plants illustrated here make up a popular herbal tincture
that was used to banish anxiety. Valerian is paired with a
mixture of more fragrant ingredients: lavender, orange peel
and ginger. Lavender is well-known for its soothing qualities
and the calming scent was considered the perfect antitode to
a worrisome mind. Ginger is packed with antioxidants which
were believed to prevent stress and an orange's peel not only
provides a more appealing flavour but also contains higher
levels of certain nutrients than its flesh.

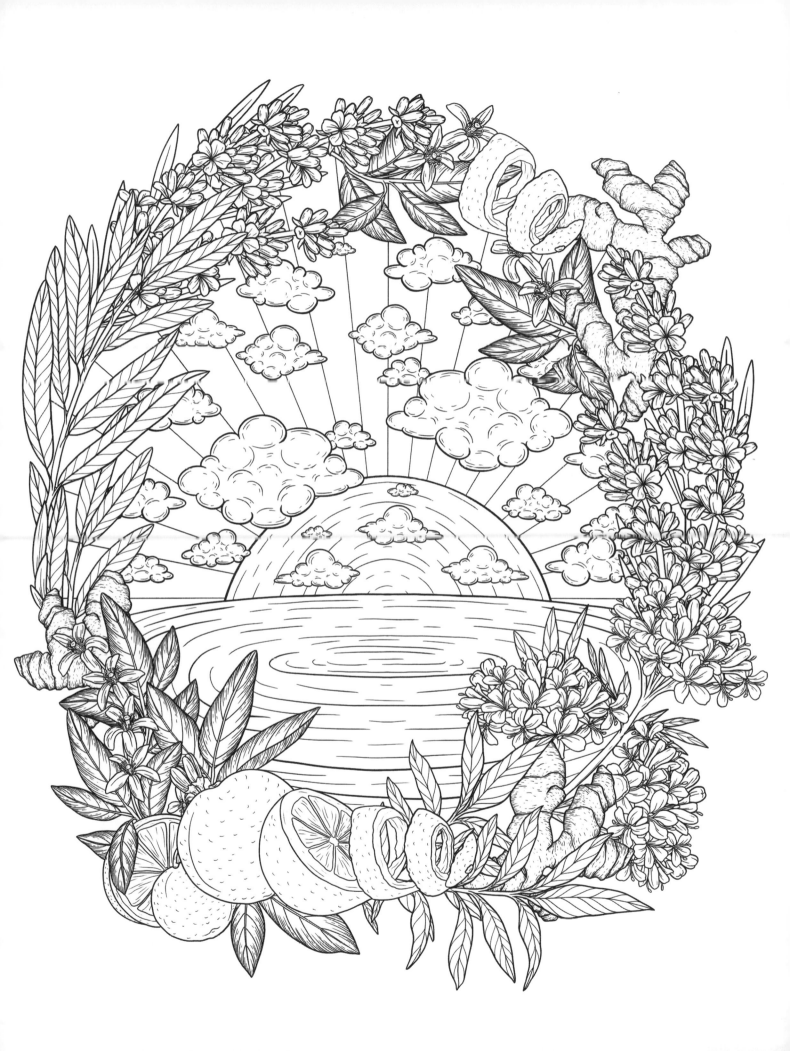

Believe in Love

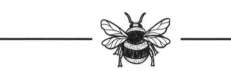

This vintage, heart-shaped perfume bottle is filled with a traditional medieval love potion – an infusion of rose petals and honey that was thought to attract love into your life if you consumed it.

Roses are synonymous with romanticism and sensuality. Their heady flavour and perfume are perfect for improving the taste and scent of potions. Honey offers the same benefits, and makes concoctions easier to swallow. It was a staple ingredient in love spells, with its sweetness expected to attract the object of the seeker's desire, and sugar-coat the ensuing relationship.

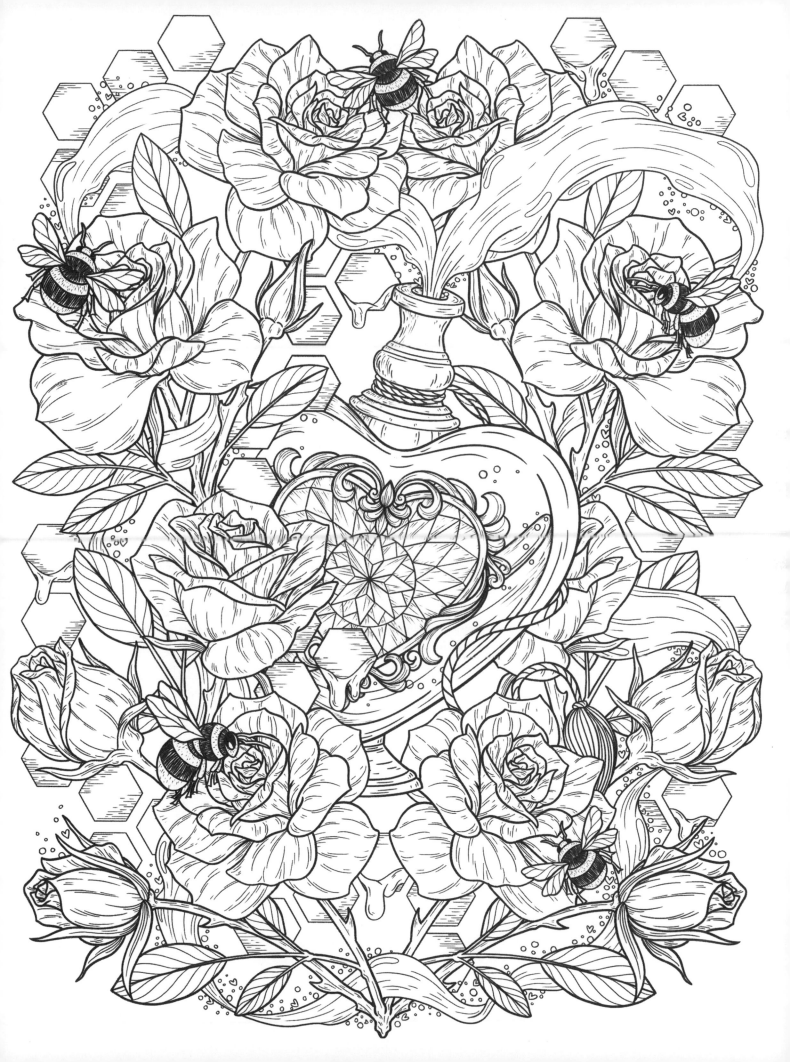

Echinacea Tincture

Echinacea plants are named for their appearance – a spiky, conical seedhead, often with purple petals. Their name comes from the Greek word 'echinos', meaning hedgehog. Despite their prickly appearance, these plants are very popular for their medicinal properties, which are believed to include boosting the immune system, relieving pain and reducing inflammation.

The plants themselves are native to North America and are believed to have been used medicinally by Indigenous peoples for over 400 years to treat infections and wounds as well as relieve headaches and soothe snake bites. A tincture was made and taken a few times throughout the day to relieve symptoms.

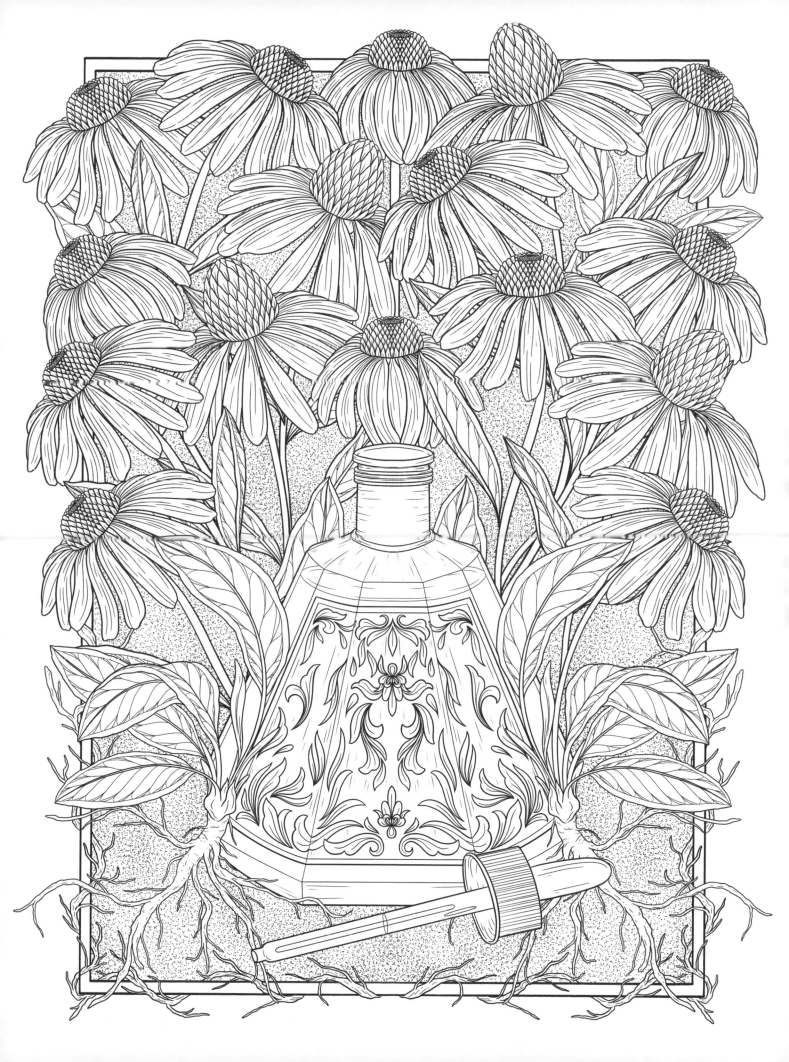

Revitalizing Soap

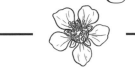

Rustic, homemade soaps can be made from a plethora
of ingredients, but this concoction features eucalyptus and
tea tree oil. The plants here are in bloom, with the distinctive
feathery flowerheads of eucalyptus and miniature flowers of
the tea tree plant, which can be pink or white. Both
of these plants are native to Australia.

Eucalyptus has many medicinal uses, which include supporting
and soothing the respiratory system. It is often used as a decongestant
when inhaled, making it a relaxing and cleansing addition to the soap.
Tea tree is considered a natural antiseptic, which helps keep skin clean
and soothes bites and blemishes. The combination of these
two plants produces a fresh-scented, cleansing soap.

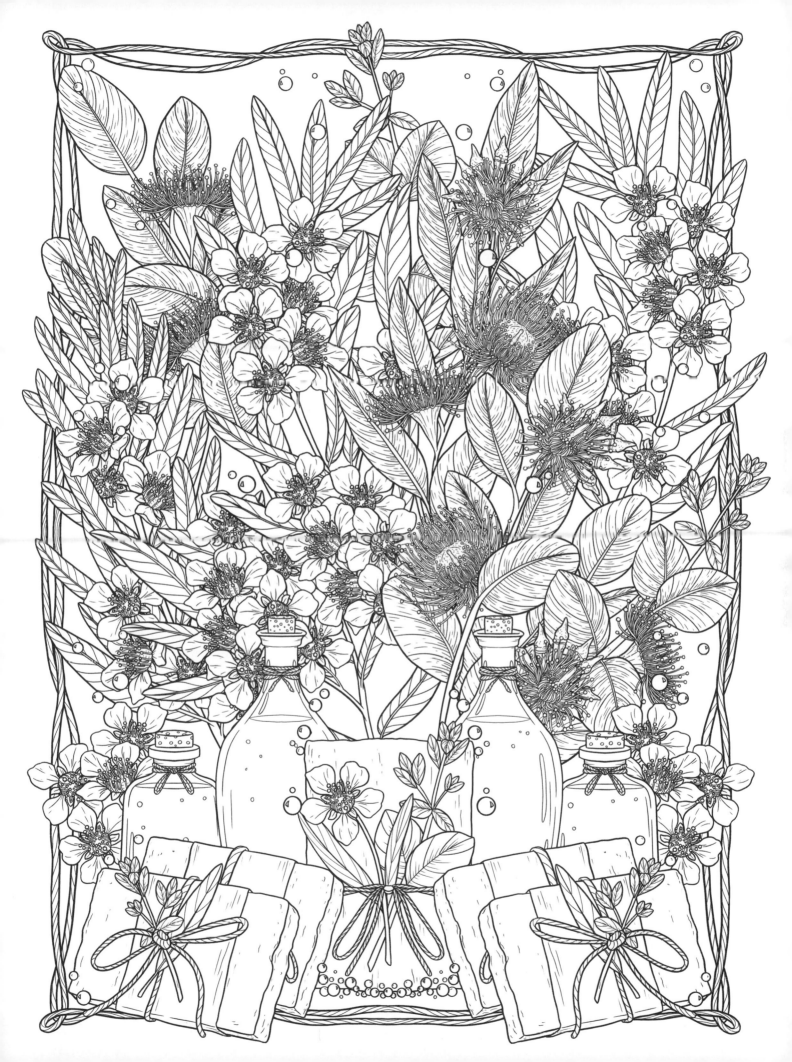

Good Luck Charm

This image features allspice and bergamot. Bergamot is a
herb that is native to North America and commonly grown to
attract pollinators. It has distinctive purple, pink or red flowers
with spiky fronds protruding from the centre of each flower head.
In herbology, it is believed to bring money, prosperity and good
sleep, while protecting people from evil and illness. Allspice is also
said to attract money and grant success in business.

This image features various forms of allspice – ground allspice, dried
berries and the leaves and flowers of the plant – which all aid compassion,
luck and healing. Pictured with golden coins, this artwork represents
the good fortune and prosperity these two herbs might bring.

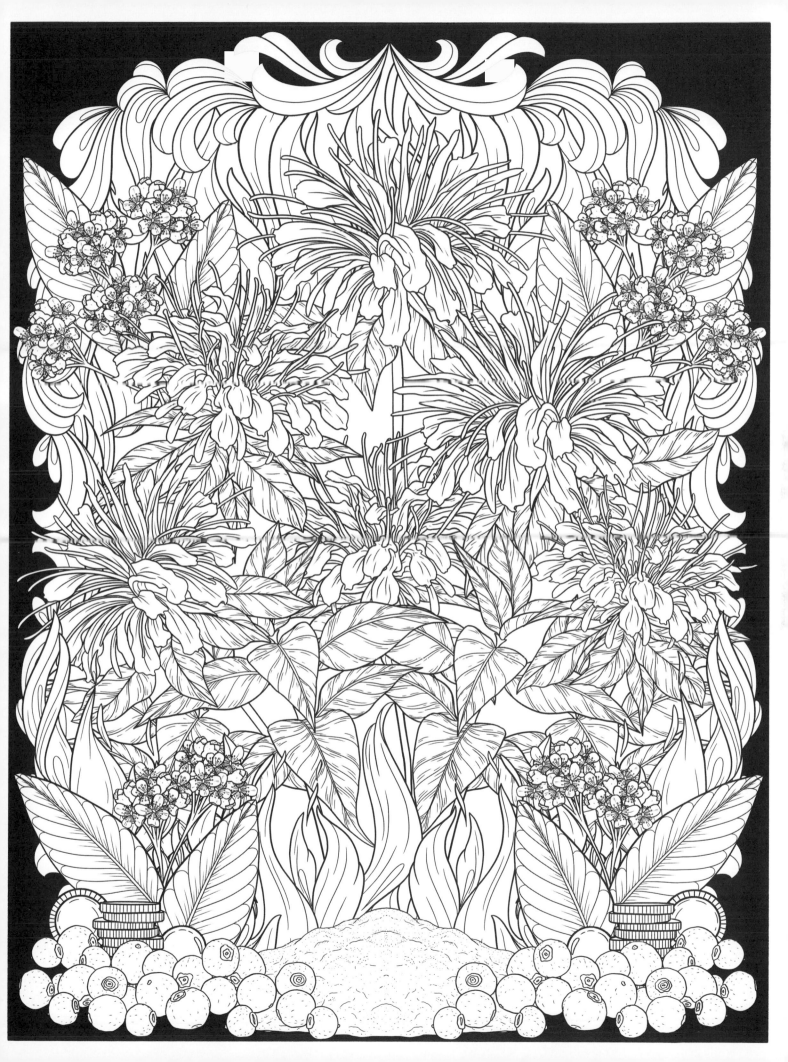

Soothing Almond

The almond tree has a rich mythology and has long been given as a gift on special occasions because of the almond's association with good fortune. It is sometimes referred to as the wakeful tree because, in its native region of the Middle East, it blossoms in January, before most other trees, and bears fruit in March. The almond itself is a nut with a brown skin, encased in a plump green shell, known as the fruit. The blossom is a delicate pale pink.

The lightly whipped moisturizer pictured here includes almond oil, which is softening and soothing, and is often added to skin products for this reason. Almonds contain an impressive number of nutrients and are packed with antioxidants. The most powerful antioxidants are found in the brown skin of the shelled almond. Evening primrose oil can be added for additional soothing qualities. Pictured here in full bloom, the evening primrose plant has long green stems and vibrant yellow flowers.

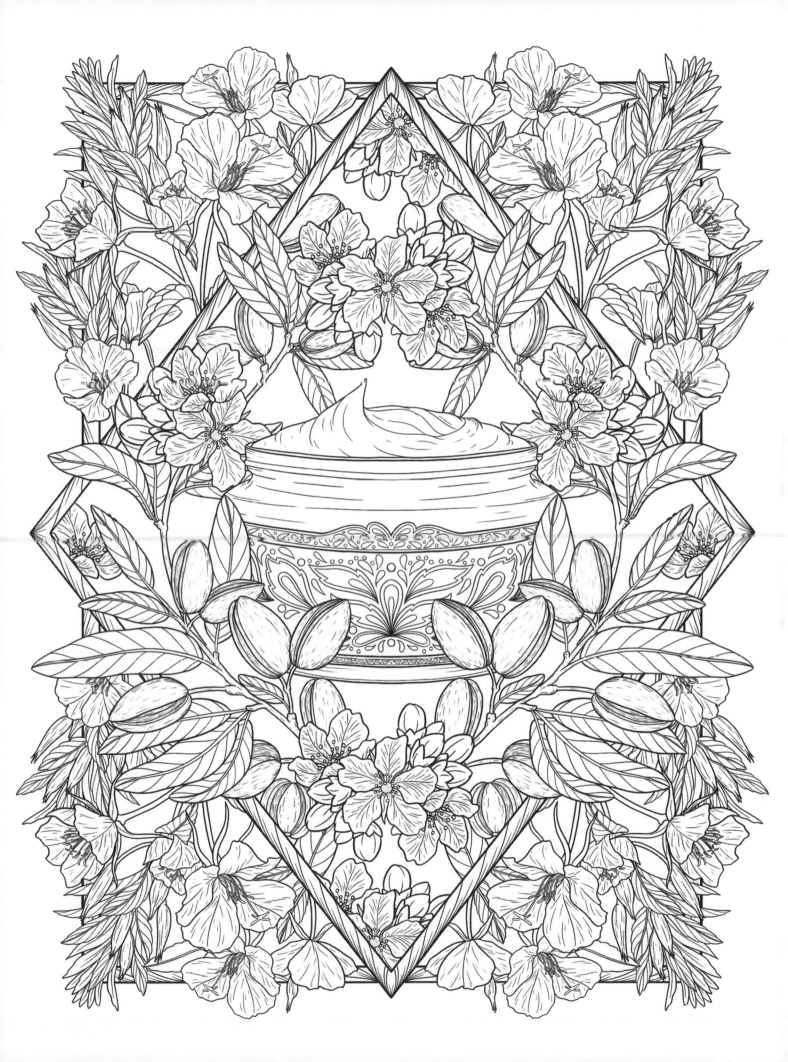

Golden Ginkgo Tree

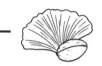

The ginkgo biloba is one of the oldest species of trees in the world – the oldest-living ginkgo tree is believed to be about 3,500 years old and fossils of ginkgo leaves have been discovered that date back 200 million years. It has very distinctive fan-shaped leaves that turn a warm golden colour in the autumn.

Ginkgo leaves and seeds have been used in traditional Chinese medicine for thousands of years. They contain many powerful antioxidants believed to reduce inflammation and open channels of energy into different organ systems, as well as improve brain function and well-being.

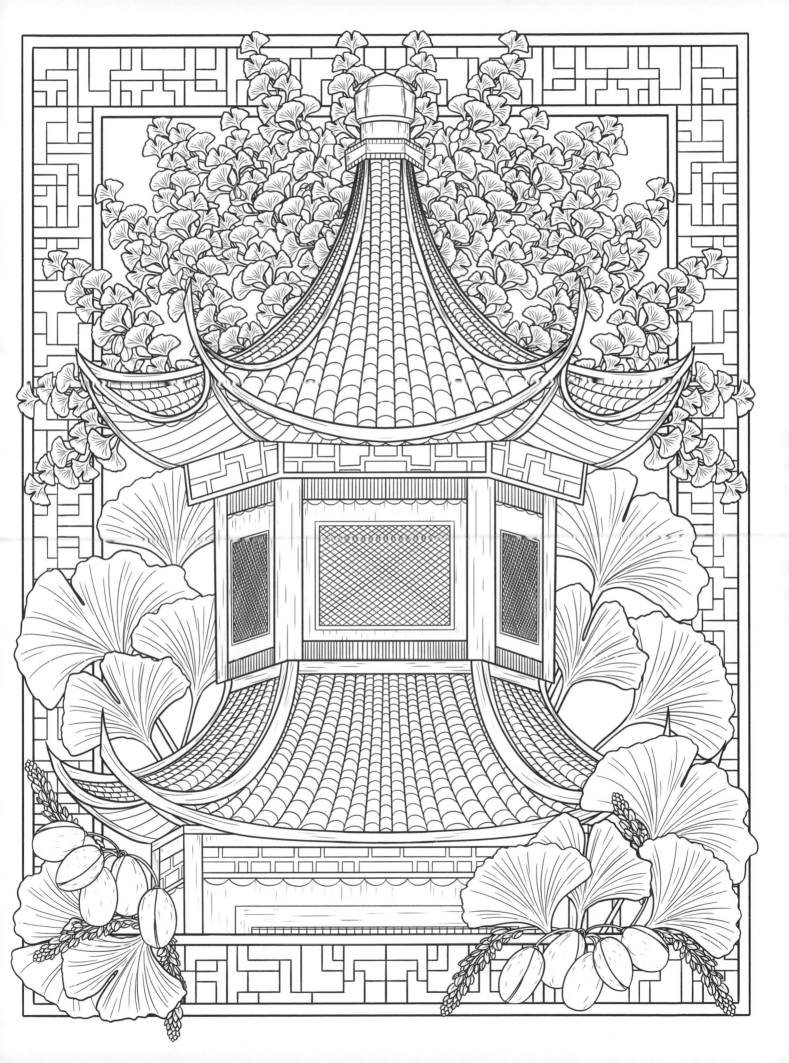

A Picture of Prosperity

This image represents a wish for prosperity, whether for
oneself or to share with others. Featuring a stained-glass Sun
with rays beaming down, a sack of gold coins and oranges
studded with cloves, it exudes positivity and good luck.

The clove tree is native to the Molucca Islands in Indonesia.
It has pale green leaves and the flowers are peachy red in colour.
In the past, the dried flower buds, known as cloves, were regularly
traded to ancient Rome and China. Cloves were so highly regarded
in these cultures that only the wealthy could afford them, hence their
association with wealth and good fortune. The tradition of gifting oranges
decorated with cloves was established by the 18th century, either at
Christmas for prosperity and protection or as fragrant
good-luck charms for the new year.

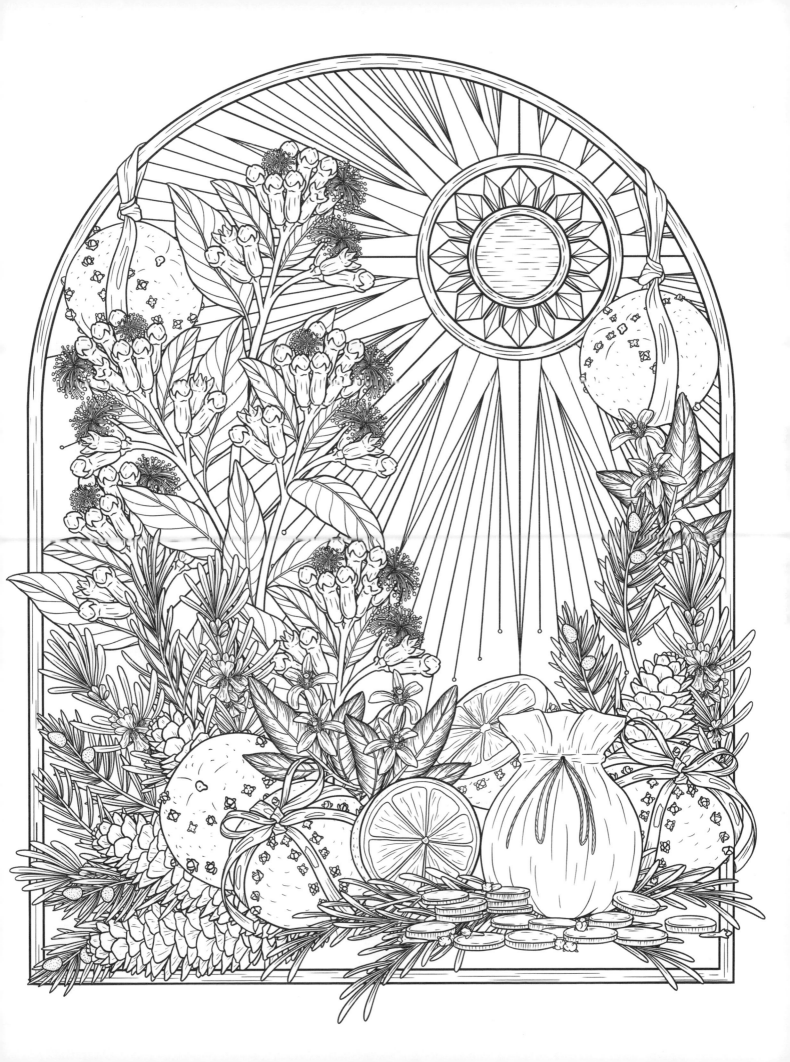

Witch's Herb

Often called the witch's herb in medieval times, rue is steeped in tradition. One of its uses in European herbal medicine has been to treat eye complaints, forming part of an eyewash to relieve strained and tired eyes. It also supposedly improved eyesight.

In addition, rue was thought to contain protective qualities that could keep evil away. Bunches of the dried herb were hung around homes for this purpose. One belief was that rue could banish a basilisk, a dreaded monster that was the subject of many folk tales. To kill a basilisk, one must place a bunch of rue in its path.

Here, a peacock is surrounded by bunches of flowering yellow rue. The peacock has historically been associated with nobility, guidance and protection. The 'eyes' on its tail feathers were believed to represent vision and watchfulness, keeping evil at bay, and there are suggestions that peacock feathers were used in potions alongside rue.

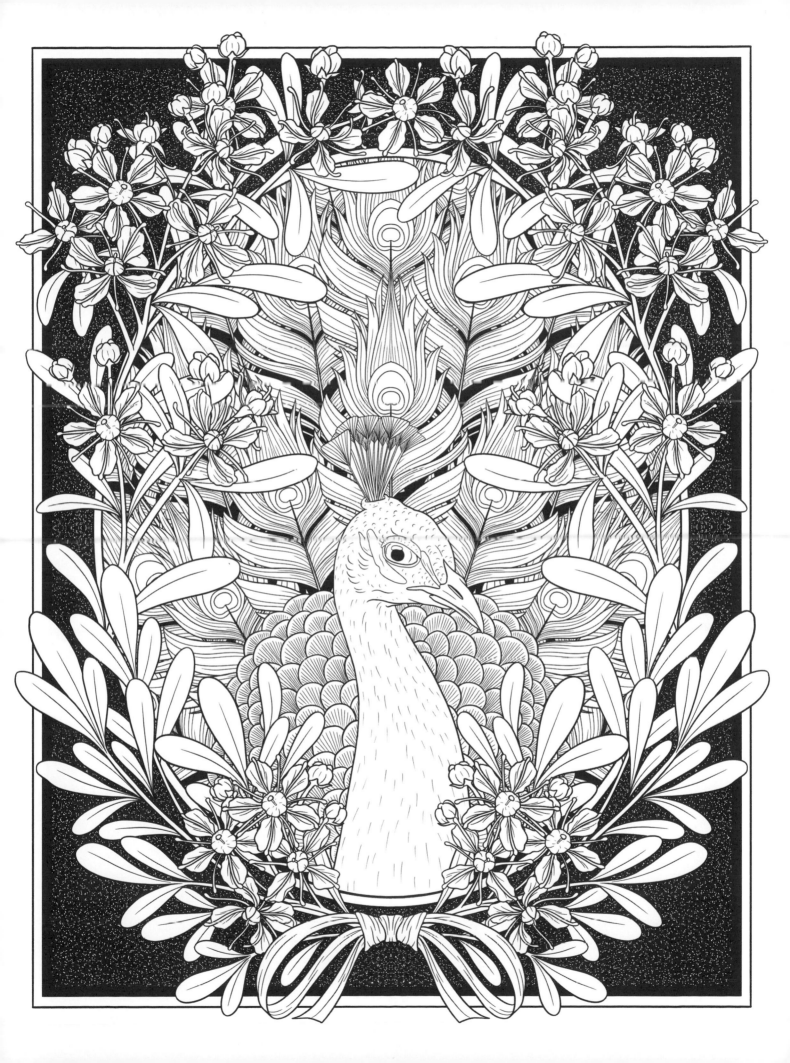

Mythical Myrrh

Myrrh is a gum resin extracted from a group of trees called *Commiphora*, native to north-east Africa. The trees flower and produce a small brown fruit. Myrrh is one of the oldest known medicines and was heavily relied on by the ancient Egyptians. It also features in traditional Chinese medicine and Ayurvedic medicine.

Myrrh was used for mouth and throat ailments, as well as in perfumes, incense and embalming. It is said to kill harmful bacteria, which explains why it was used as part of the embalming process, as it slows decay while also having a pleasant smell. More modern-day uses include aiding skin conditions and treating wounds and infections. Myrrh supports oral health, protecting against gum disease and mouth ulcers, with the plant extract featuring in some natural mouthwashes and toothpastes.

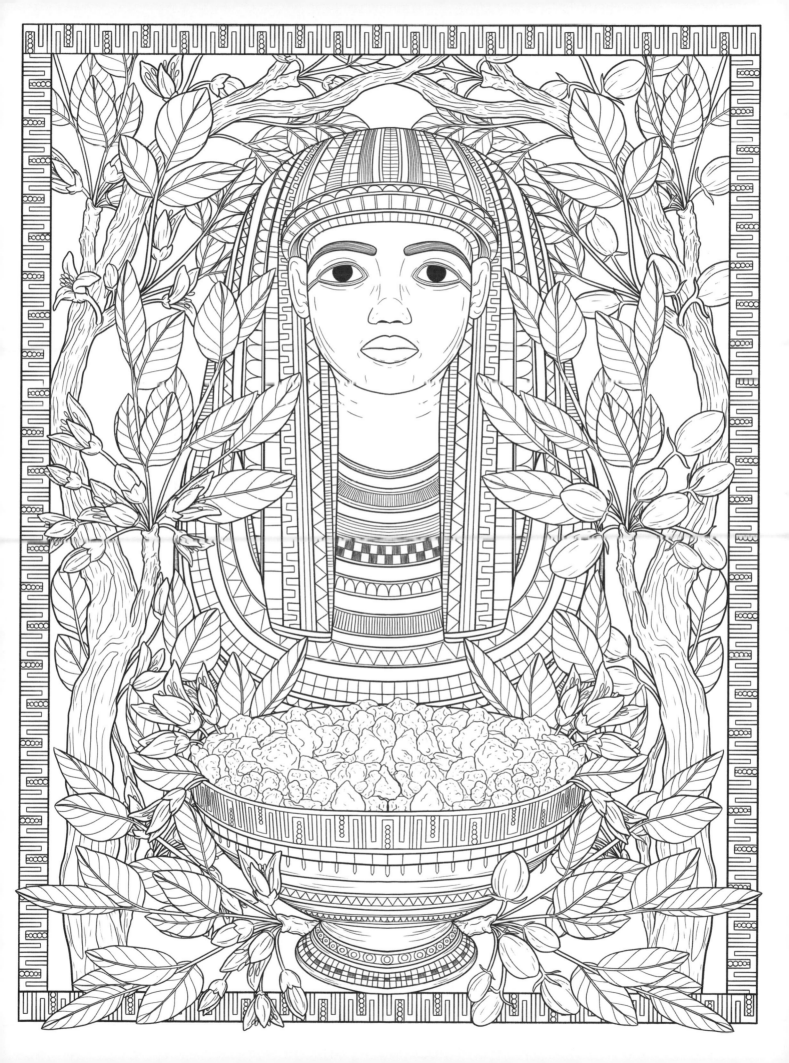

Home Charm

This berry bouquet is made of holly and mistletoe. Both were believed to ward off evil and were used to prevent malign spirits from entering the home. Holly trees were planted near houses to offer protection against lightning, and the prickly leaves were thought to keep witches at bay. Mistletoe was revered by the Druids and considered sacred because it grew on oak trees, which is where the word Druid comes from – the Celtic name for the oak tree is 'Duir'.

This home charm features both holly, with its waxy green leaves and red berries, and mistletoe, with pale green leaves and white berries. The bunch is tied with a ribbon with a small charm adorning it. In the middle is a waxwing, a bird that loves to feast on holly and mistletoe berries come winter. Waxwings have warm red feathers on their heads and bright splashes of yellow on their wings and tail.

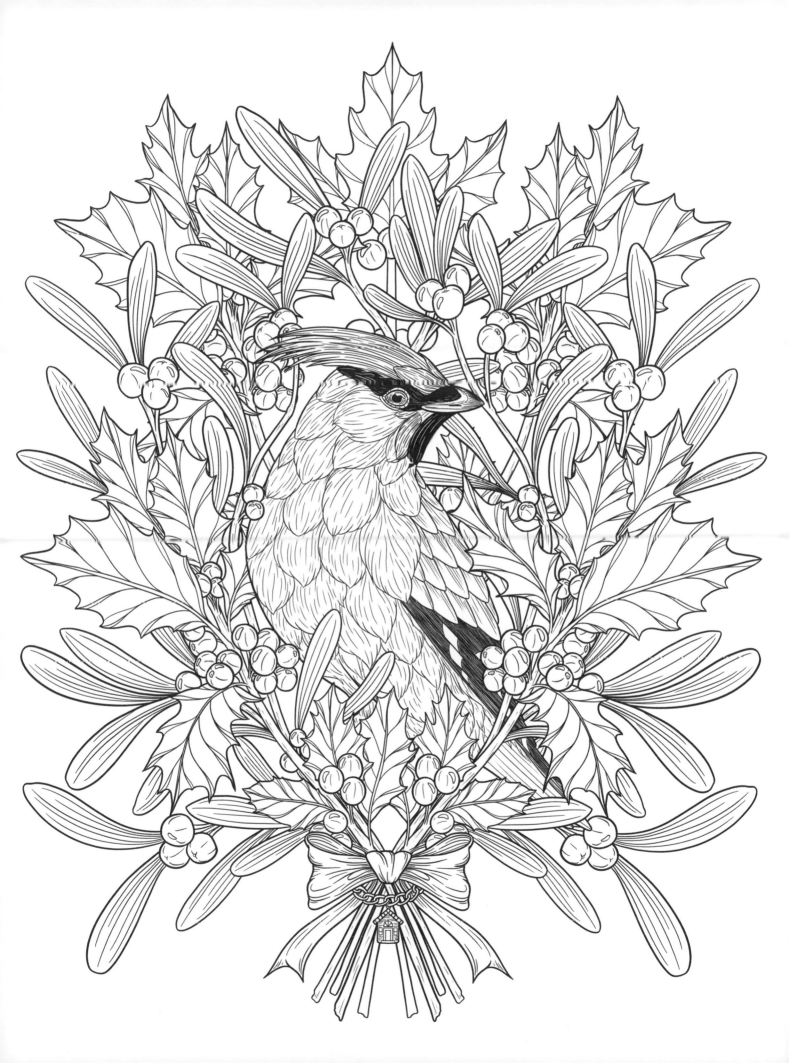

Balm for Bruises

This basket of beautiful blooms contains powerful plants
that have been used medicinally for many years.

Arnica, comfrey leaves and yarrow have traditionally been
used to soothe bruises, aches and strained muscles. Arnica is
a pretty plant with a yellow flower that grows most commonly in
Europe and America. It has been used as a remedy for arthritis, as well
as to treat pain and swelling. Comfrey is well known for its distinctive
long, slender leaves and black-skinned roots. It has been used
traditionally in Japan for over 2,000 years, primarily to treat
bruises, sprains and inflammation. Yarrow is a delicate plant with
lots of small flowers that bloom in clusters. It is also considered
to act as an anti-inflammatory when applied to the skin.

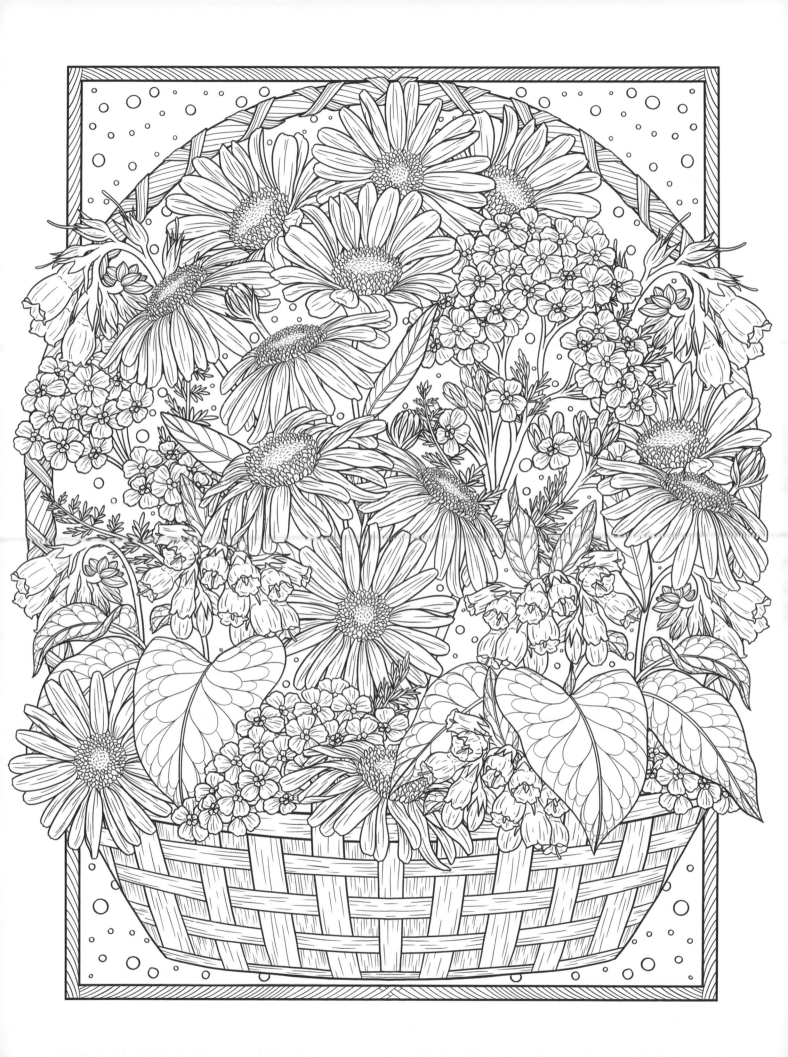

Spiritual Cinnamon

Cinnamon has many medicinal uses and has been revered
for its properties for thousands of years. Cinnamon sticks are made
from the inner bark of the cinnamon tree, which can then be ground
down to a powder. The tall cinnamon trees have luscious green
leaves and small buds that produce tiny flowers.

Cinnamon is loaded with antioxidants and has been used as
a remedy for colds because of its warming qualities. It is said to have
anti-inflammatory properties, which would also contribute to cold relief.
As well as these uses, cinnamon has strong connections with solar magic
and spirituality. It is renowned for its powers of healing, protection
and prosperity, which are alluded to here by the crystal ball.

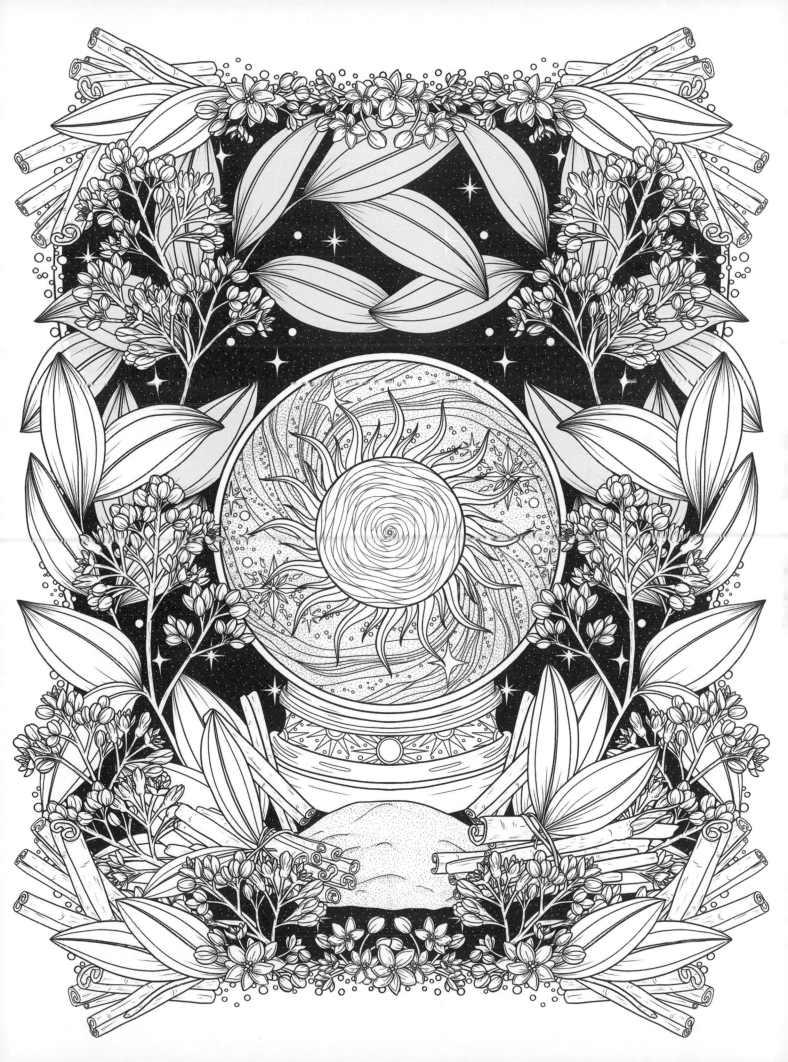

Acai Bowl

Acai bowls are a popular breakfast dish made from crushed
acai berries and other fruits. Acai berries are a 'superfruit' and are
the fruit of the acai palm, which grows in Central and South American
rainforests. The dark purple acai berries have a very short shelf life,
so they are often exported as purée, powder or juice. The reason these
berries are so popular is because of their nutritional value. They are
packed with antioxidants, are believed to boost brain function
and some think they can improve cholesterol levels.

Shown here in a decorative bowl, acai berries are accompanied
by kiwi, banana and strawberries, and surrounded by the
palm leaves and branches from the acai tree.

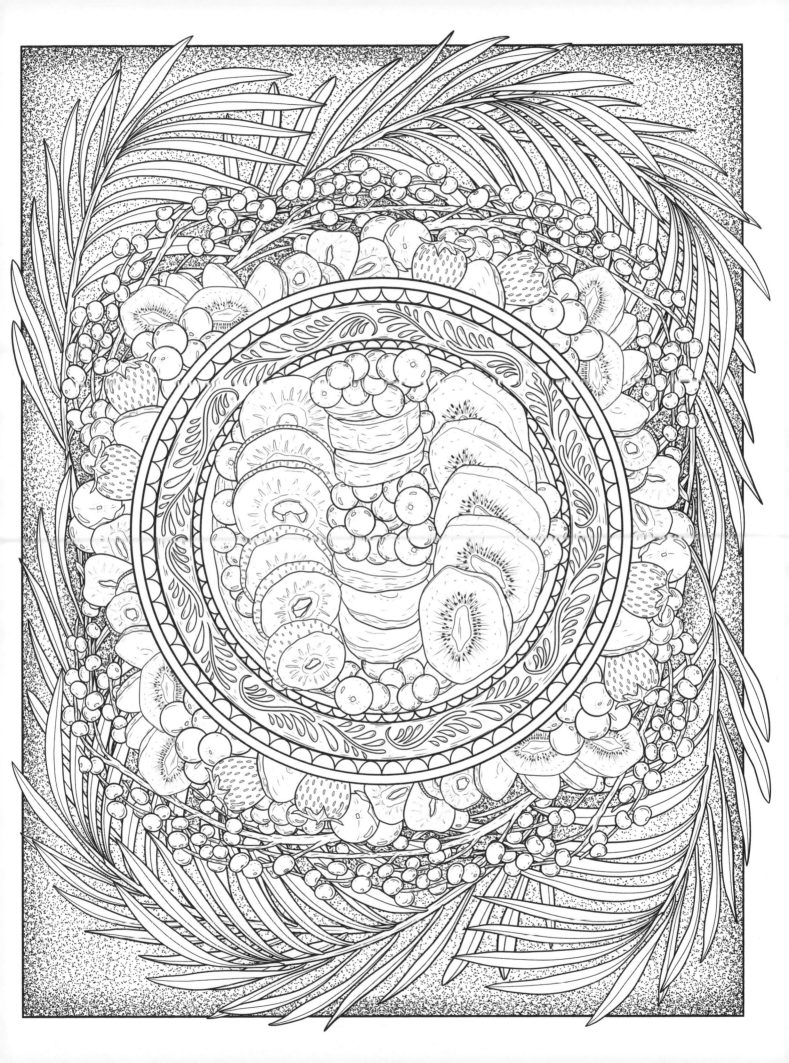

A Cure for Colds

Nepeta cataria, or catnip, as it is more commonly known,
is native to Europe and is part of the mint family. It has dark
green leaves and small flowers that are often purple or white.
It is said to stimulate sweating and has therefore been used
to treat fevers, colds and flu. Tonics can be sweetened
with elderflower and honey to enhance flavour.

It is probably best known today for its association with
cats. The dried leaves are often used as filling for cat toys,
as the leaves and stems contain nepetalactone, an oil
that stimulates a sensory response in most cats and
can trigger a period of excitable behaviour in them.

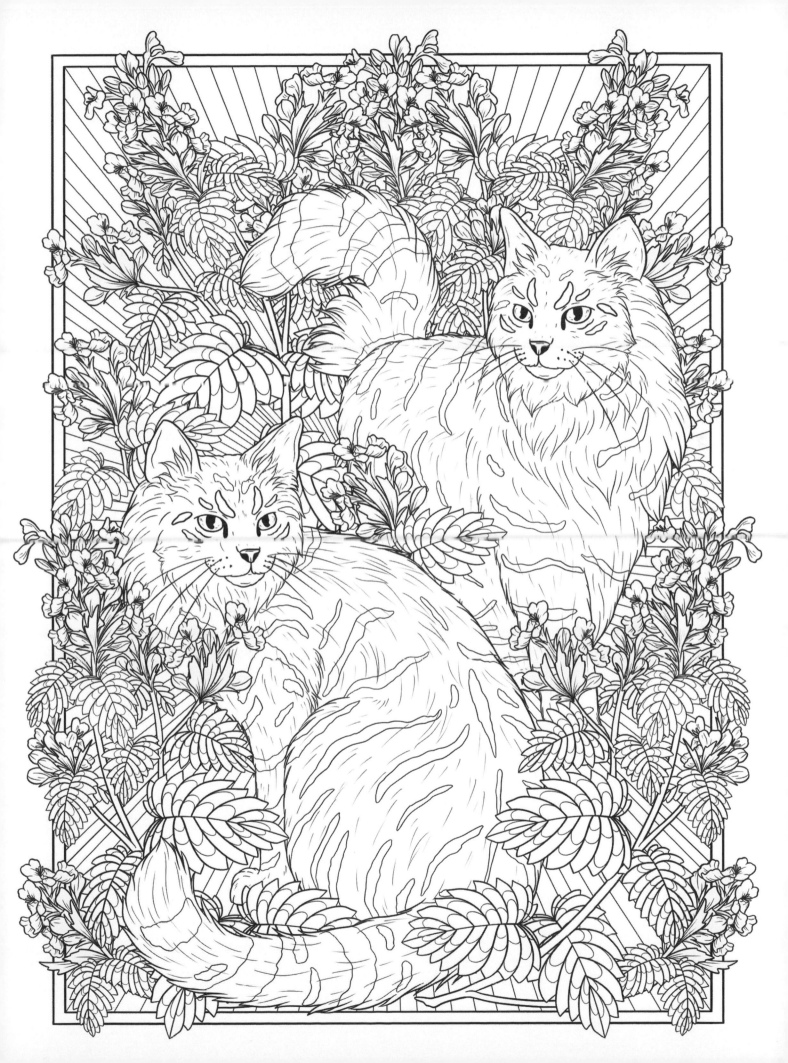

Easing Joints

Turmeric is an important spice in Ayurvedic medicine. It has been
used for thousands of years to soothe inflammation, and in recent years
has become a popular homeopathic remedy for easing arthritis symptoms.
The long, fresh green leaves surround a distinctive purple flower. The
part of turmeric that is consumed is the bulb that grows under
the ground, which is a warm, sunny orange colour.

One of the reasons turmeric is so revered is because it contains
a compound called curcumin. This is an active ingredient that has
powerful anti-inflammatory and antioxidant effects, which can alleviate
sore joints. Black pepper, which is pictured here alongside the turmeric,
is known to help the body absorb curcumin. Presented in a traditional
Indian spice box are little bowls of peppercorns and ground turmeric,
surrounded by luscious turmeric plants and vibrant
green peppercorns growing in clusters.

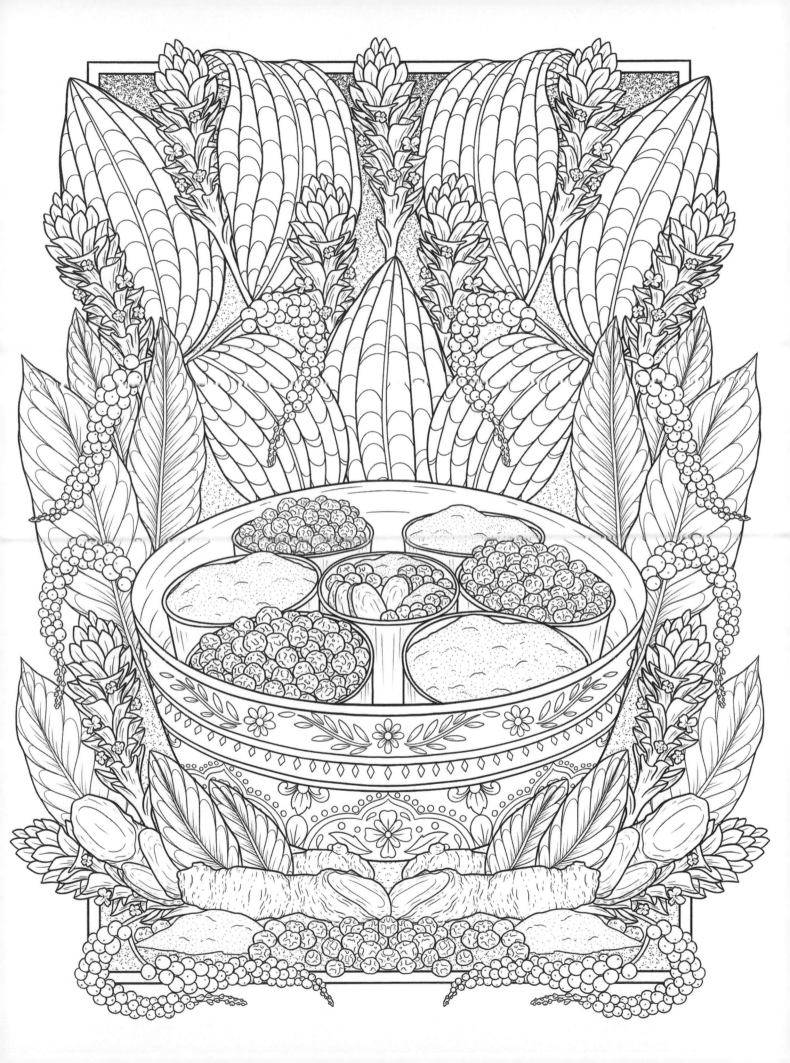

Natural Skin Reviver

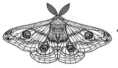

This pretty pattern, featuring both flora and fauna, is full of delicate blooms to colour. It is made up of meadowsweet and witch hazel, with bumble bees and emperor moths resting on the flowers.

Meadowsweet is a herb that has been used in traditional medicine for centuries. It is a member of the rose family and has small flowers that are usually creamy yellow or white. It contains salicylates and tannins, which are believed to have anti-inflammatory effects in the body.

Witch hazel also has lots of naturally occuring anti-inflammatory properties and antioxidants, and has long been used in skin and hair products. It has distinctive flowers with long fronds that are often a golden yellow colour. Mixing these two plants together produces a soothing and energizing treatment for the skin that has a sweet scent.

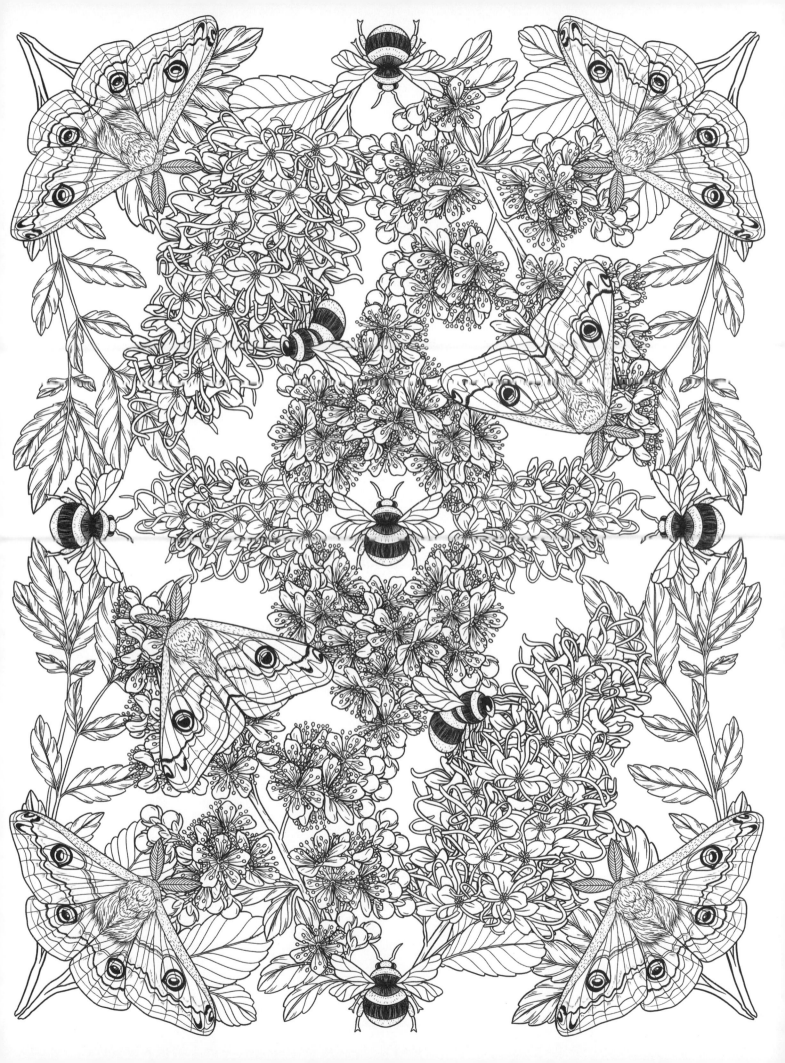

Toothache Tonic

The neem tree belongs to the mahogany family. It has small, fragrant flowers and yellow-green fruit. The neem is valued as a medicinal plant and has long been used in Ayurvedic and folk medicine, as well as cosmetics. Almost every part of the tree, from the seeds and bark to the leaves, are valued for their antibacterial and antifungal properties.

Here, the neem is accompanied by a clove tree, with its distinctive clove-shaped flowers in full bloom. A tincture to relieve toothache was made by heating water, neem bark and cloves together until boiling. Once the liquid had cooled, it was applied directly to the site of pain. A male and female black-naped oriole adorn the illustration as these black-and-yellow birds are known to feast on the fruits of the neem tree.

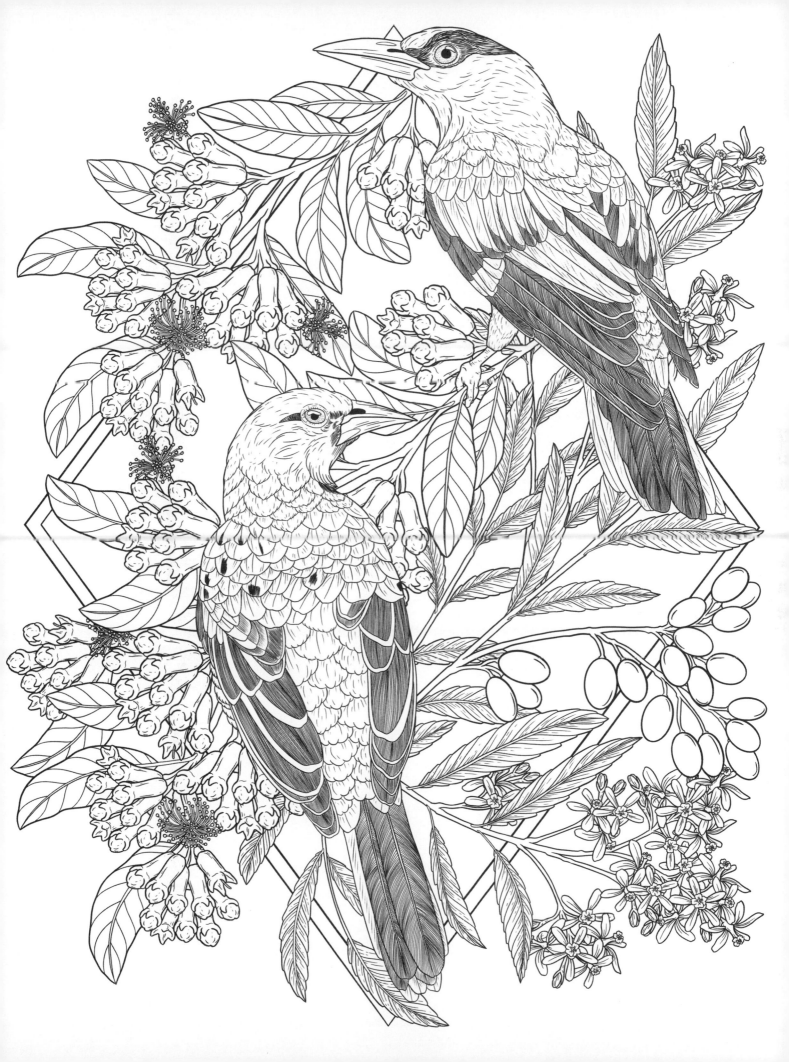

Healing Geranium

The beautiful geranium comes in a range of hues, from pinks and purples to reds and oranges, and is a favourite of pollinators. This pretty bloom has long been revered and it has a strong association with happiness and healing.

Some varieties of the geranium were thought to keep snakes at bay and wild geranium roots were often used as a cure for sore throats. One popular potion was taken to soothe a broken heart. It was made by steeping the fresh geranium flowers in water and boiling them for ten minutes. The brew was then strained, a spoonful of honey was added and pale pink rose petals were sprinkled on top.

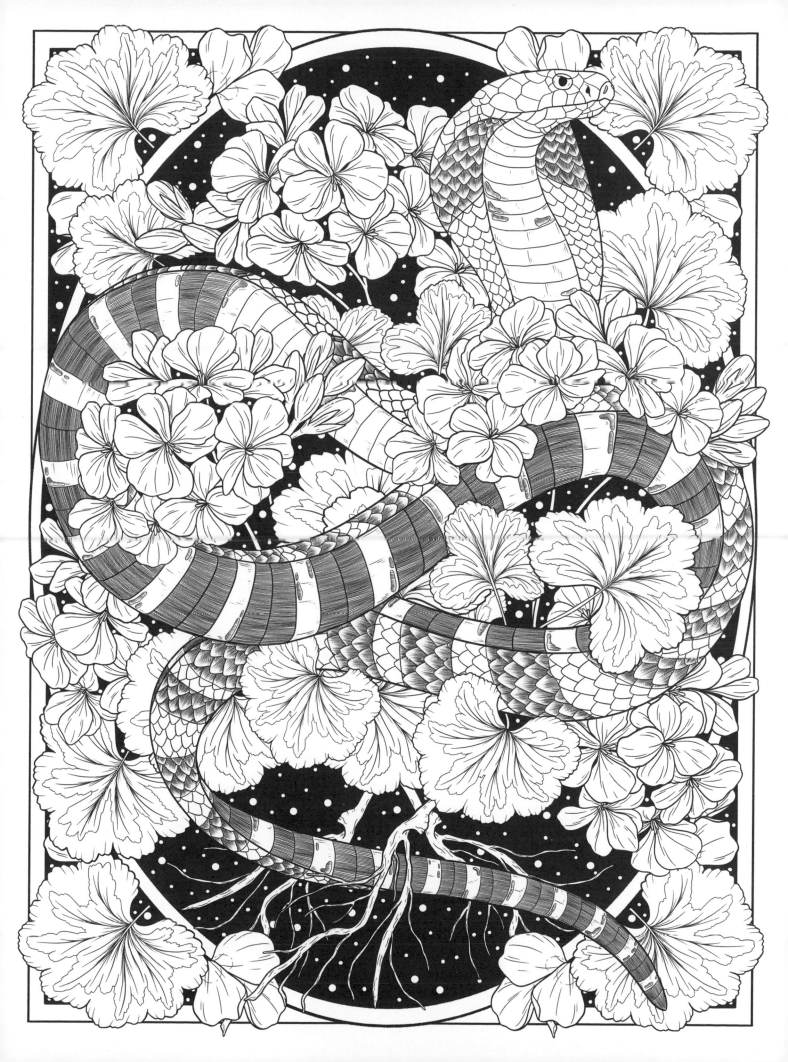

Sweet Superberries

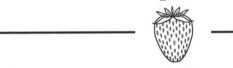

Superfoods are nutrient-rich, often plant-based foods that
are believed to be beneficial for health and well-being. They are
often packed with vitamins, minerals and antioxidants.

This beautiful bowl of berries and surrounding plants is made
up of strawberries, blueberries and cranberries. Although they all
have lots of nutritional benefits blueberries, in particular, have high
levels of vitamin K. Strawberries are one of the best sources of vitamin
C and cranberries are known to have high levels of flavonoids.
These bright and colourful berries can be eaten as they are,
or made into juices, conserves or teas.

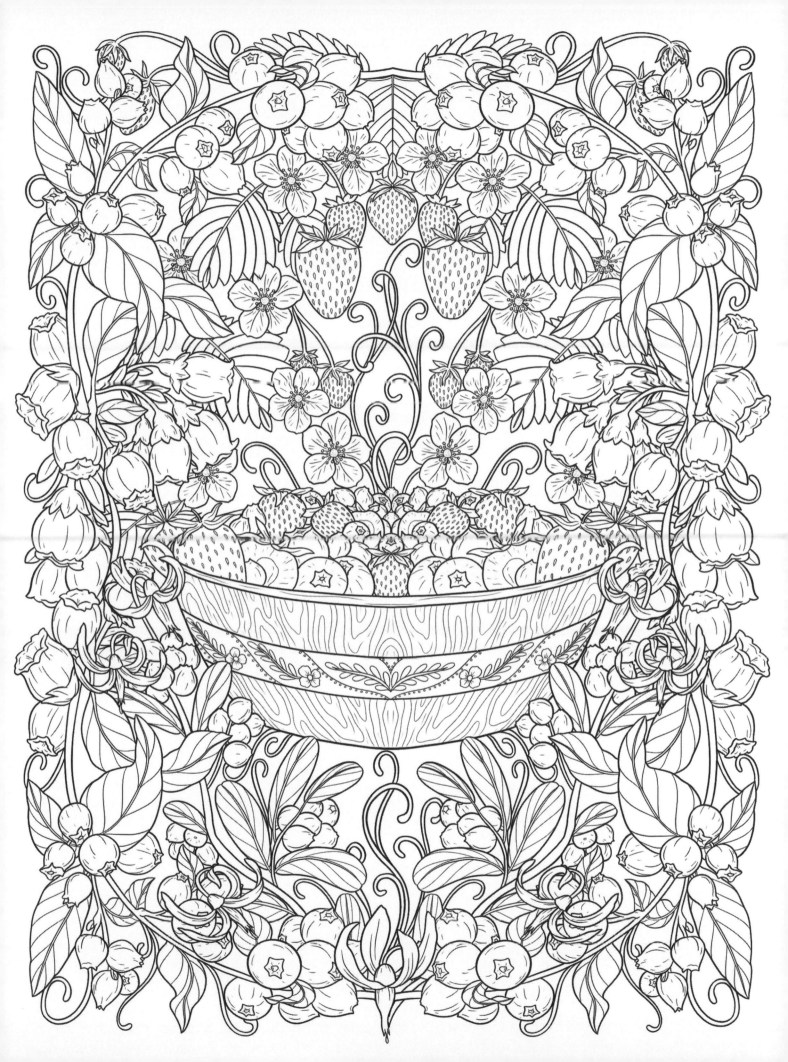

Fire Cider Tonic

Fire cider tonic has been used in traditional medicine to cure colds and banish the flu for many years. The name itself was coined by a herbalist in the 1970s, but many variations were created before then and have been created since. The recipe combines apple cider vinegar with other natural ingredients, which are then left to stew before being strained and decanted. The tonic can then either be sipped or added to other brews.

Exact recipes vary, but this image features garlic, horseradish, onion, ginger, turmeric, peppercorns, chilli, cinnamon and rosemary. These ingredients are prized for their anti-inflammatory, antioxidant and antimicrobial properties. Lemon and honey can be added as well as to enhance the flavour and sweetness.

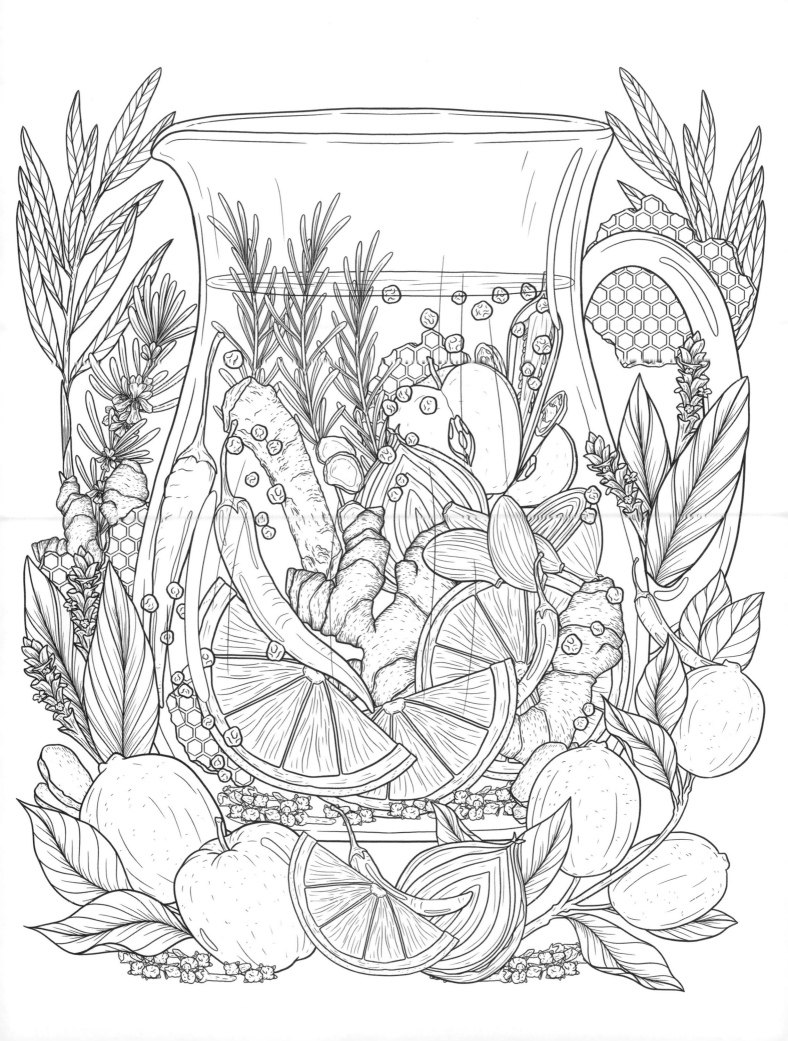

Herbal Headdress

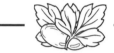

In ancient times, it was believed that if you carried an olive leaf with you, you'd keep headaches at bay. Olives are naturally anti-inflammatory and have long been synonymous with peace and harbouring soothing properties. The oil extract from the plant is still used today in hair and skin products. A popular herbal compress and headache cure involved binding olive leaves and parsley leaves to the forehead.

This herbal headdress is made up of olive branches with dark green leaves, white-and-yellow flowers and rich black olives alongside parsley and bound with a ribbon. It encircles an old, twisted olive tree. A white dove symbolizes the peace associated with olive plants and the soothing properties of this compress.

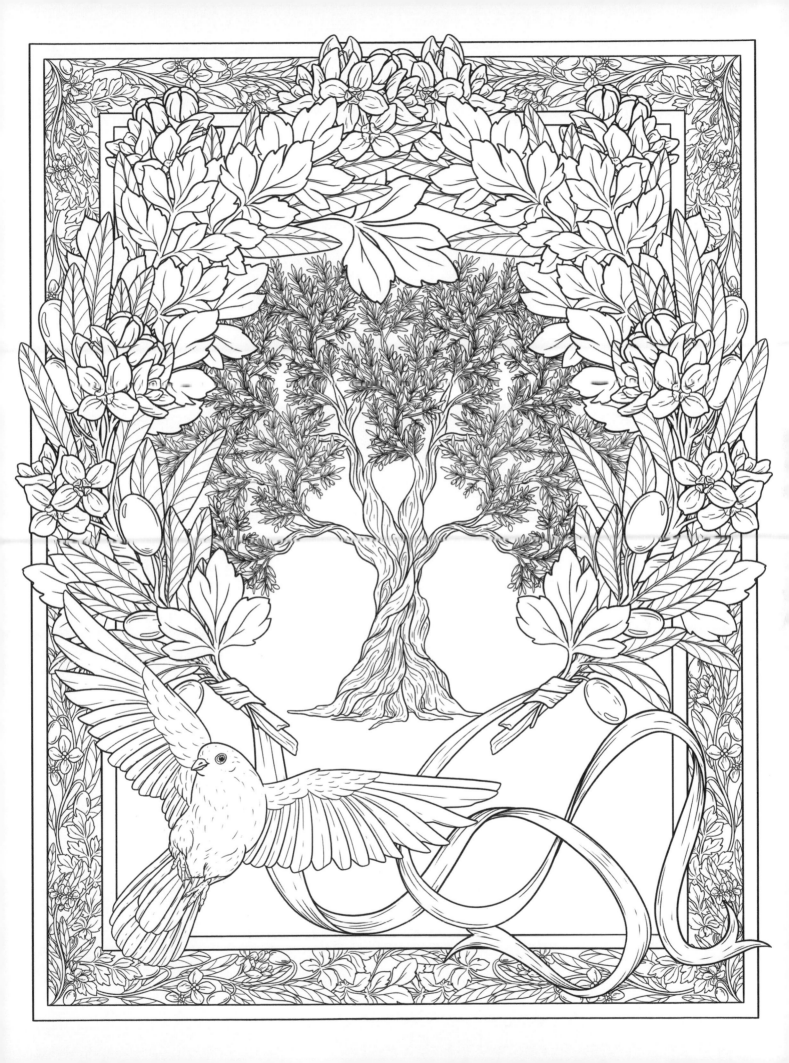

Wildflower Mead

Mead is a traditional alcoholic beverage made with honey,
water and yeast, that has been in existance for many thousands
of years, with some Chinese pottery dating from 7000 BCE showing
traces of mead fermentation. It was a popular drink throughout history,
with the Vikings, Mayans and ancient Egyptians, Greeks and Romans
creating their own concoctions. The Greeks called mead 'nectar of
the gods' and the Vikings would drink it on their way into battle.

This image depicts a wildflower mead, featuring honeycomb, orange,
lavender, wild violets, dandelion, golden raisins and a scoop of yeast.
These delicate ingredients surround a wooden tankard with
a carving of a honeybee emblem etched on to it.

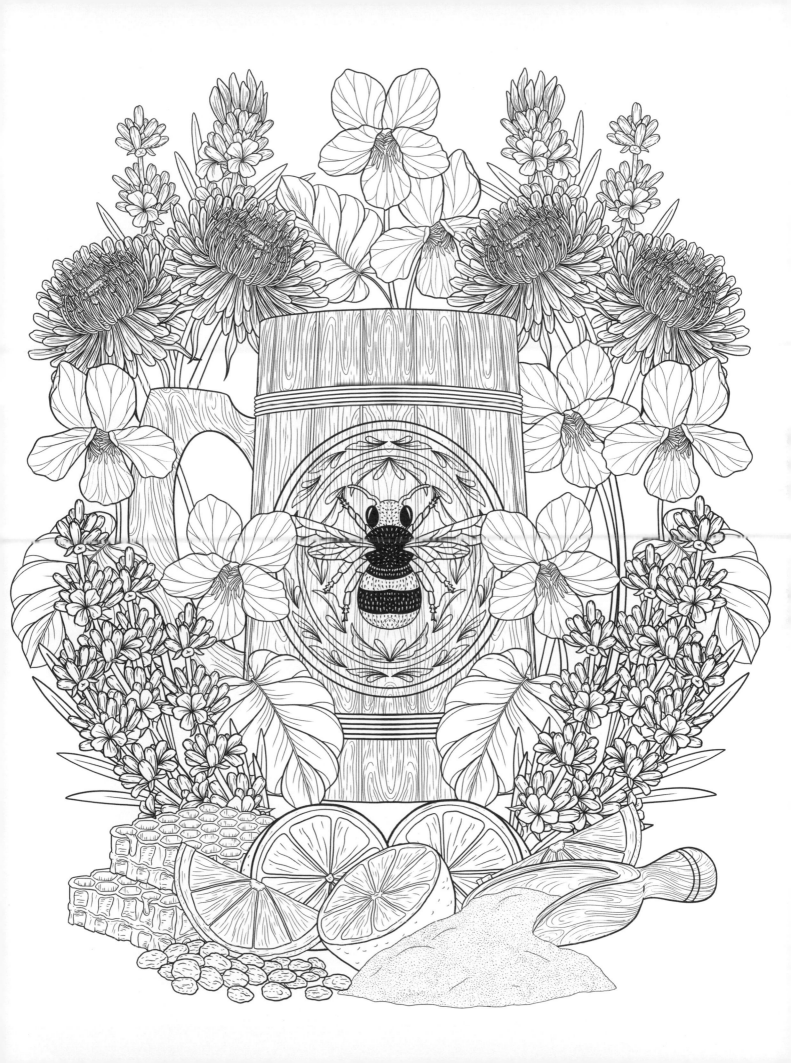

Face Cleanser

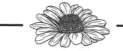

This bouquet of fragrant and colourful herbs and flowers is made up of lemon balm, chamomile, roses, calendula, comfrey leaf, rosemary and sage, with lemons adorning the borders. These ingredients make for a cleansing and energizing facewash.

Lemon balm is rich in antioxidants and anti-inflammatory properties, which protects skin and reduces redness. It also has a pleasant, lemony aromatic scent. Chamomile is soothing and helps to relieve itchy and painful skin. Rose has moisturizing qualities and is rich in vitamins, helpful for softening skin and easing wrinkles. Calendula is antimicrobial and helps to heal wounds and also relieves inflammation. Comfrey leaf can decrease pain and swelling, and helps to rejuvenate cells. Rosemary helps to stimulate the circulatory system and also adds a delicate scent, while sage aids in tightening and toning tissue. The acid of the lemon is an excellent cleanser and contains antioxidants that nourish the skin.

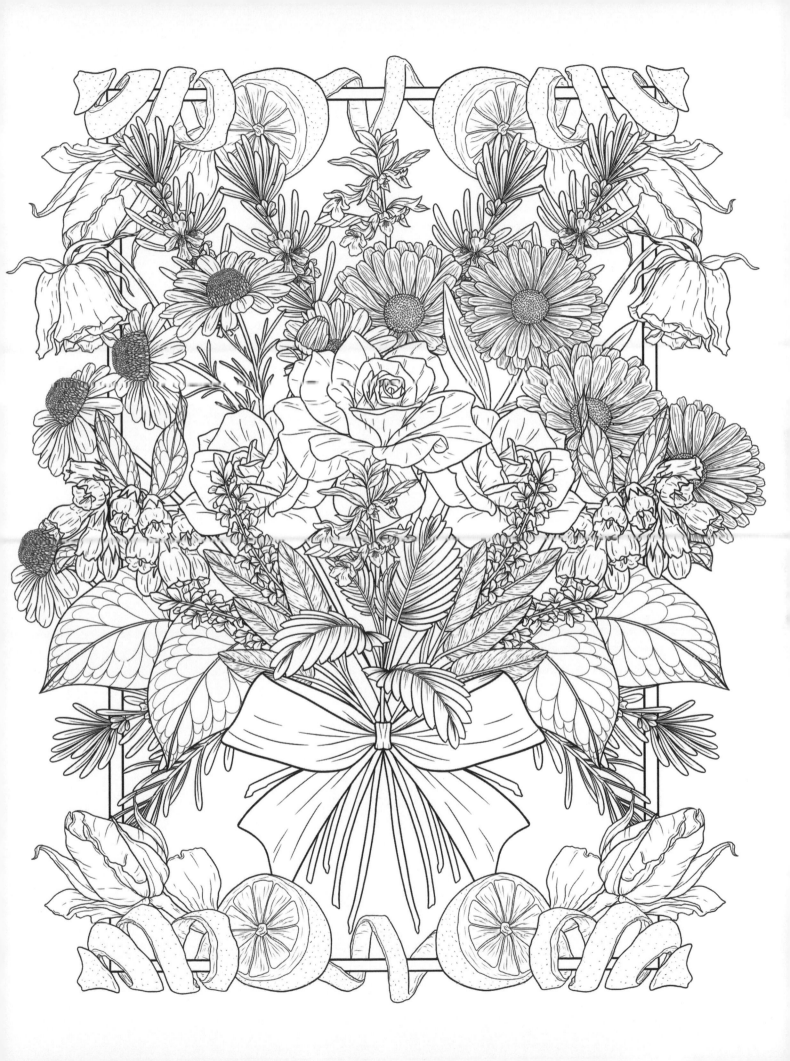

Soothing Tonic

This tonic features plants that have soothing properties and can help to relieve sore throats. A jar of sweet honey is surrounded by eucalyptus, liquorice and marshmallow, all pictured in flower. The feathery flowers of eucalyptus come in a range of colours, from vibrant reds to pinks. Liquorice flowers are purple and marshmallow flowers are white with a deep purple centre.

Eucalyptus is widely used as a natural remedy for colds and is commonly used in cold and cough products to help relieve congestion and headaches. The use of liquorice in a medical capacity dates back to ancient Egypt. It too is used to relieve coughs and is believed to help with bacterial and viral infections. It is also believed to soothe sore throats and has the additional benefit of providing a sweeter flavour to the products it's used in. Marshmallow root is deemed to relieve coughs and colds, particularly a dry cough and an irritated throat. Likewise, honey is a well-known natural remedy for sore throats, as it can ease irritation as well as add a pleasing flavour.

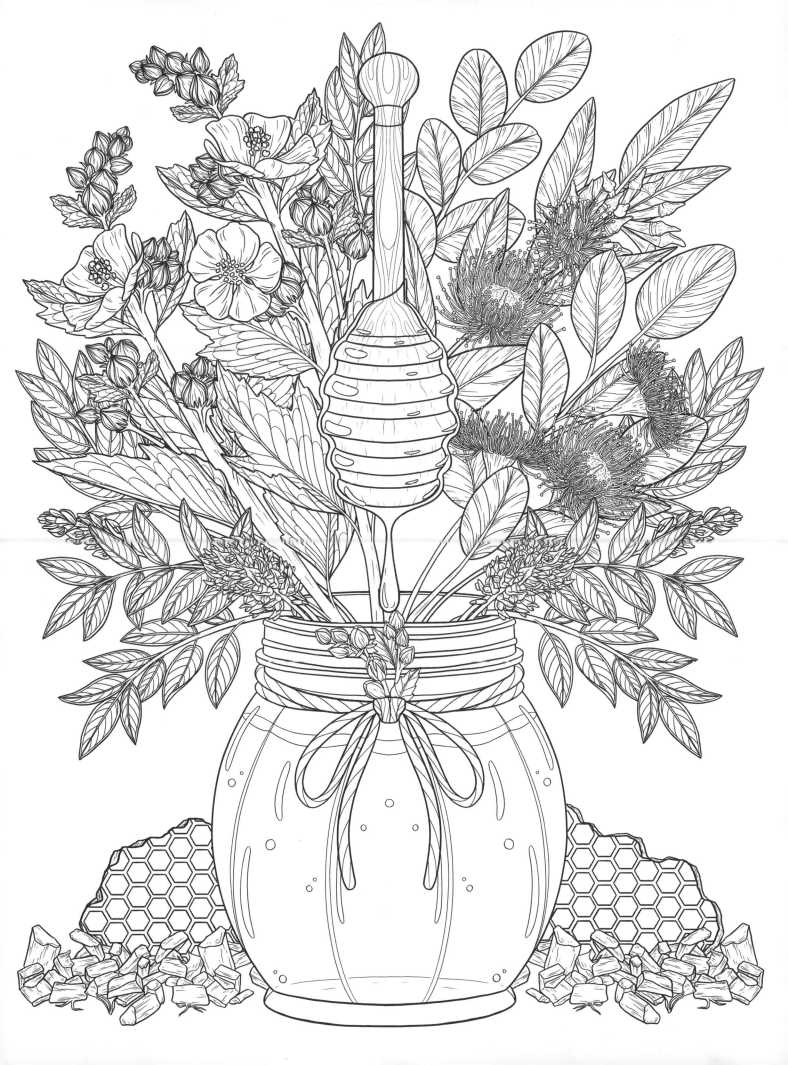

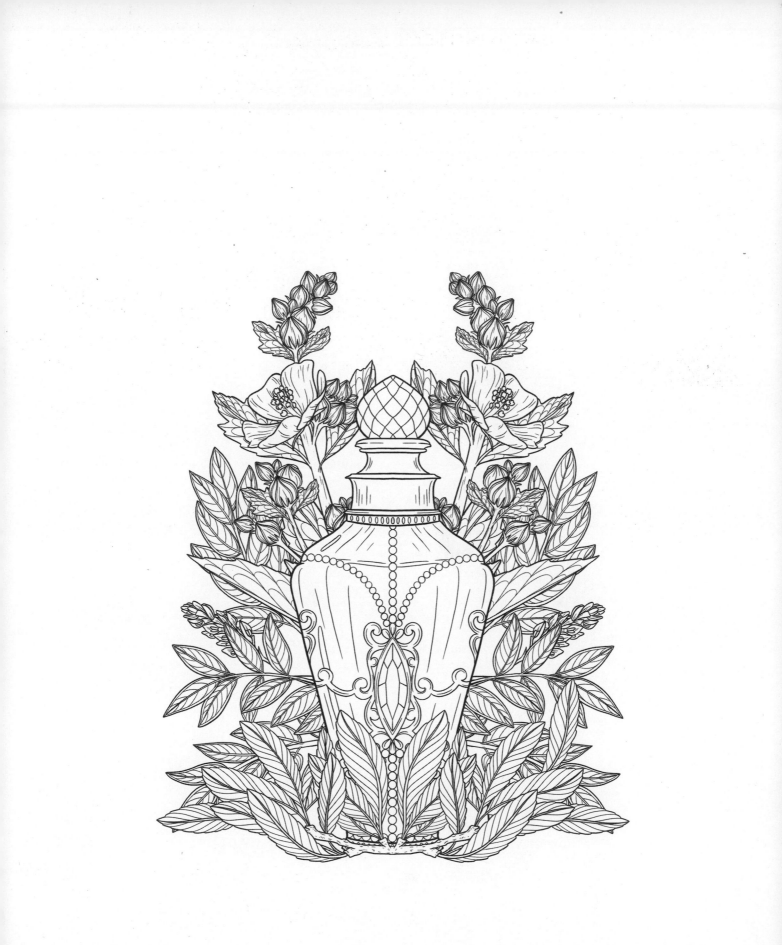